Low
Fat
Pizza
Recipes

"Delicious Low Fat Pizza Recipes for
Flavourful, Healthy Meals"

Jennifer Bailey

Low Fat Pizza Recipes

Disclaimer

Please keep in mind that the content in this book is solely for educational purposes. The information offered here is said to be reliable and trustworthy. The author makes no implication or intends to offer any warranty of accuracy for particular individual cases. Before beginning any diet or lifestyle habits, it is recommended that you contact a knowledgeable practitioner, such as your doctor. This book's material should not be utilized in place of expert counsel or professional guidance.
The author, publisher, and distributor expressly disclaim all liability, loss, damage, or danger incurred by persons who rely on the information in this book, whether directly or indirectly.
All intellectual property rights are retained. This book's information should not be replicated in any way, mechanically, electronically, photocopying, or by any other methods accessible

Table of Contents

Chapter 1: Introduction to Low Fat Pizza

In recent years, pizza has earned a somewhat undeserved reputation as a guilty pleasure, often associated with high fat, high calorie, and less-than-healthy ingredients. However, with a little creativity and some smart ingredient substitutions, pizza can absolutely be a part of a balanced and nutritious diet. This chapter serves as a gateway into the world of low fat pizza, exploring the benefits and offering tips for crafting delicious, healthier versions of this beloved dish.

Understanding the Benefits of Low Fat Pizza

Low fat pizza offers a multitude of benefits for those looking to enjoy this classic comfort food without compromising their health goals. Here are some key advantages:

1. **Reduced Caloric Intake**: By opting for low fat ingredients and lighter toppings, you can significantly decrease the calorie content of your pizza, making it a more waistline-friendly option.

2. **Heart Health**: Traditional pizza often contains high levels of saturated fat, which can contribute to heart disease. Choosing low fat alternatives can help lower your intake of unhealthy fats and support cardiovascular health.

3. **Weight Management**: Incorporating low fat pizza into your meal rotation can be a helpful strategy for those looking to manage their weight. With fewer calories and less fat, it's easier to stay within your daily calorie goals while still enjoying a satisfying meal.

4. **Improved Nutrition Profile**: By loading your pizza with nutrient-rich toppings like vegetables and lean proteins, you can boost its nutritional value, packing it with vitamins, minerals, and antioxidants.

5. **Satisfying Cravings**: Let's face it—pizza is delicious, and sometimes nothing else will satisfy a craving for cheesy, savory goodness. Low fat pizza

allows you to indulge in this comfort food favorite without derailing your diet.

Tips for Making Delicious Low Fat Pizza

Creating a tasty low fat pizza is all about making smart ingredient choices and employing clever cooking techniques. Here are some tips to help you whip up a healthier pie:

1. **Choose Whole Grain Crusts**: Opt for whole wheat or multigrain pizza crusts to increase the fiber content of your pizza and add extra nutrients.

2. **Load Up on Veggies**: Vegetables are not only low in fat and calories but also packed with essential nutrients. Load your pizza with colorful veggies like bell peppers, mushrooms, spinach, onions, and tomatoes for added flavor and nutrition.

3. **Go Easy on the Cheese**: While cheese adds richness and flavor to pizza, it's also a significant source of fat and

Chapter 2: Low fat pizza crusts

1. Whole Wheat Herb Crust Pizza

Intro: This whole wheat herb crust pizza offers a nutritious twist on a classic favorite. The combination of whole wheat flour and fragrant herbs creates a flavorful base for your favorite toppings.

Total Time: 1 hour 30 minutes (including resting time)

Servings: Makes one 12-inch pizza crust

Ingredients:
- 1 cup whole wheat flour
- 1 teaspoon active dry yeast
- 1/2 teaspoon sugar
- 1/2 teaspoon salt
- 1 tablespoon olive oil
- 1/2 cup warm water
- 1 teaspoon dried Italian herbs (such as oregano, basil, and thyme)

Directions:

1. In a small bowl, combine the warm water, sugar, and yeast. Let it sit for 5-10 minutes until frothy.
2. In a large mixing bowl, combine the whole wheat flour, salt, dried herbs, and olive oil. Add the yeast mixture and mix until a dough forms.
3. Knead the dough on a lightly floured surface for about 5 minutes, until smooth and elastic.
4. Place the dough in a lightly oiled bowl, cover with a clean kitchen towel, and let it rise in a warm place for about 1 hour, or until doubled in size.
5. Preheat your oven to 425°F (220°C). Roll out the dough on a lightly floured surface to your desired thickness.
6. Transfer the rolled-out dough to a pizza stone or baking sheet lined with parchment paper.
7. Add your favorite toppings, then bake in the preheated oven for 15-20 minutes, or until the crust is golden brown and crispy.
8. Slice and serve hot.

Nutritional Information (per serving):
- Calories: 180 kcal
- Fat: 4g
- Carbohydrates: 30g
- Fiber: 4g
- Protein: 6g

2. Cauliflower and Flaxseed Crust Pizza

Intro: This cauliflower and flaxseed crust pizza is a gluten-free and low carb alternative to traditional pizza crusts. It's packed with fiber and nutrients while still delivering that satisfying pizza experience.

Total Time: 45 minutes

Servings: Makes one 10-inch pizza crust

Ingredients:
- 1 small head cauliflower, riced (about 2 cups)
- 2 tablespoons ground flaxseed
- 1/4 cup grated Parmesan cheese
- 1/2 teaspoon dried oregano
- 1/2 teaspoon garlic powder

- 1/4 teaspoon salt
- 1 egg

Directions:

1. Preheat your oven to 400°F (200°C). Line a baking sheet with parchment paper.
2. Place the riced cauliflower in a microwave-safe bowl and microwave on high for 4-5 minutes, or until softened. Allow to cool slightly.
3. Place the cooked cauliflower in a clean kitchen towel and squeeze out as much moisture as possible.
4. In a large mixing bowl, combine the cauliflower, ground flaxseed, Parmesan cheese, oregano, garlic powder, salt, and egg. Mix until well combined.
5. Transfer the cauliflower mixture to the prepared baking sheet and spread it out into a circle, about 1/4 inch thick.
6. Bake in the preheated oven for 20-25 minutes, or until the crust is golden brown and firm.
7. Remove from the oven and let cool slightly before adding your favorite toppings.

8. Return the pizza to the oven and bake for an additional 10-15 minutes, or until the toppings are heated through and the cheese is melted.
9. Slice and serve hot.

Nutritional Information (per serving):
- Calories: 120 kcal
- Fat: 6g
- Carbohydrates: 9g
- Fiber: 5g
- Protein: 8g

3. Quinoa Crust Mediterranean Pizza

Intro: This quinoa crust Mediterranean pizza offers a unique and nutritious twist on traditional pizza. Packed with protein and fiber from quinoa, and topped with Mediterranean-inspired ingredients, it's a delicious and satisfying meal.

Total Time: 50 minutes

Servings: Makes one 12-inch pizza crust

Ingredients:
- 1 cup cooked quinoa, cooled

- 1 egg
- 1/4 cup grated Parmesan cheese
- 1/2 teaspoon dried basil
- 1/2 teaspoon dried oregano
- 1/4 teaspoon garlic powder
- Salt and pepper to taste

Directions:

1. Preheat your oven to 425°F (220°C). Line a baking sheet with parchment paper.
2. In a large mixing bowl, combine the cooked quinoa, egg, Parmesan cheese, basil, oregano, garlic powder, salt, and pepper. Mix until well combined.
3. Transfer the quinoa mixture to the prepared baking sheet and spread it out into a circle, about 1/4 inch thick.
4. Bake in the preheated oven for 15-20 minutes, or until the crust is set and lightly golden brown.
5. Remove from the oven and let cool slightly before adding your favorite toppings.
6. Return the pizza to the oven and bake for an additional 10-15 minutes, or until

the toppings are heated through and the cheese is melted.

7. Slice and serve hot.

Nutritional Information (per serving):

- Calories: 150 kcal
- Fat: 5g
- Carbohydrates: 18g
- Fiber: 2g
- Protein: 8g

4. Sweet Potato and Oat Crust Pizza

Intro: This sweet potato and oat crust pizza offers a wholesome and gluten-free alternative to traditional pizza crusts. The combination of sweet potatoes and oats creates a hearty and flavorful base that pairs perfectly with a variety of toppings.

Total Time: 50 minutes

Servings: Makes one 10-inch pizza crust

Ingredients:

- 1 cup cooked mashed sweet potato
- 1 cup rolled oats
- 1 egg

- 1/4 teaspoon garlic powder
- 1/4 teaspoon dried thyme
- Salt and pepper to taste

Directions:

1. Preheat your oven to 400°F (200°C). Line a baking sheet with parchment paper.
2. In a food processor, combine the cooked mashed sweet potato, rolled oats, egg, garlic powder, dried thyme, salt, and pepper. Pulse until a dough forms.
3. Transfer the dough to the prepared baking sheet and spread it out into a circle, about 1/4 inch thick.
4. Bake in the preheated oven for 20-25 minutes, or until the crust is set and lightly golden brown.
5. Remove from the oven and let cool slightly before adding your favorite toppings.
6. Return the pizza to the oven and bake for an additional 10-15 minutes, or until the toppings are heated through and the cheese is melted.
7. Slice and serve hot.

Nutritional Information (per serving):
- Calories: 130 kcal
- Fat: 3g
- Carbohydrates: 22g
- Fiber: 3g
- Protein: 5g

5. Almond Flour Thin Crust Pizza

Intro: This almond flour thin crust pizza offers a low carb and gluten-free option for pizza lovers. With the nutty flavor of almond flour and a crispy texture, it's a delicious base for your favorite toppings.

Total Time: 30 minutes

Servings: Makes one 12-inch pizza crust

Ingredients:
- 1 1/2 cups almond flour
- 1 egg
- 1/2 teaspoon garlic powder
- 1/2 teaspoon dried basil
- 1/4 teaspoon salt
- 1/4 teaspoon black pepper

Directions:

1. Preheat your oven to 400°F (200°C). Line a baking sheet with parchment paper.
2. In a large mixing bowl, combine the almond flour, egg, garlic powder, dried basil, salt, and black pepper. Mix until a dough forms.
3. Transfer the dough to the prepared baking sheet and use your hands to press it out into a thin circle, about 1/8 inch thick.
4. Bake in the preheated oven for 15-20 minutes, or until the crust is golden brown and crispy.
5. Remove from the oven and let cool slightly before adding your favorite toppings.
6. Return the pizza to the oven and bake for an additional 10-15 minutes, or until the toppings are heated through and the cheese is melted.
7. Slice and serve hot.

Nutritional Information (per serving):

- Calories: 180 kcal
- Fat: 14g
- Carbohydrates: 7g
- Fiber: 3g
- Protein: 8g

6. Brown Rice and Chia Seed Crust Pizza

Intro: This brown rice and chia seed crust pizza is a nutritious and gluten-free alternative to traditional pizza crusts. Packed with fiber and omega-3 fatty acids, it offers a wholesome base for your favorite toppings.

Total Time: 50 minutes

Servings: Makes one 12-inch pizza crust

Ingredients:
- 1 cup cooked brown rice, cooled
- 2 tablespoons chia seeds
- 1 egg
- 1/4 cup grated Parmesan cheese
- 1/2 teaspoon dried rosemary
- 1/2 teaspoon garlic powder

- Salt and pepper to taste

Directions:
1. Preheat your oven to 400°F (200°C). Line a baking sheet with parchment paper.
2. In a food processor, combine the cooked brown rice, chia seeds, egg, Parmesan cheese, dried rosemary, garlic powder, salt, and pepper. Pulse until a dough forms.
3. Transfer the dough to the prepared baking sheet and spread it out into a circle, about 1/4 inch thick.
4. Bake in the preheated oven for 25-30 minutes, or until the crust is set and lightly golden brown.
5. Remove from the oven and let cool slightly before adding your favorite toppings.
6. Return the pizza to the oven and bake for an additional 10-15 minutes, or until the toppings are heated through and the cheese is melted.
7. Slice and serve hot.

Nutritional Information (per serving):
- Calories: 160 kcal
- Fat: 6g
- Carbohydrates: 20g
- Fiber: 3g
- Protein: 7g

7. Zucchini and Parmesan Crust Pizza

Intro: This zucchini and Parmesan crust pizza is a low carb and gluten-free option that's bursting with flavor. With the freshness of zucchini and the nuttiness of Parmesan cheese, it's a delightful twist on traditional pizza crusts.

Total Time: 45 minutes

Servings: Makes one 10-inch pizza crust

Ingredients:
- 2 cups grated zucchini, squeezed to remove excess moisture
- 1/2 cup grated Parmesan cheese
- 1 egg
- 1/4 teaspoon dried basil
- 1/4 teaspoon dried oregano

- 1/4 teaspoon garlic powder
- Salt and pepper to taste

Directions:

1. Preheat your oven to 425°F (220°C). Line a baking sheet with parchment paper.
2. In a large mixing bowl, combine the grated zucchini, Parmesan cheese, egg, dried basil, dried oregano, garlic powder, salt, and pepper. Mix until well combined.
3. Transfer the zucchini mixture to the prepared baking sheet and spread it out into a circle, about 1/4 inch thick.
4. Bake in the preheated oven for 20-25 minutes, or until the crust is set and lightly golden brown.
5. Remove from the oven and let cool slightly before adding your favorite toppings.
6. Return the pizza to the oven and bake for an additional 10-15 minutes, or until the toppings are heated through and the cheese is melted.
7. Slice and serve hot.

Nutritional Information (per serving):
- Calories: 140 kcal
- Fat: 8g
- Carbohydrates: 6g
- Fiber: 1g
- Protein: 10g

8. Polenta and Herbs Crust Pizza

Intro: This polenta and herbs crust pizza offers a unique and flavorful base for your favorite toppings. With the creamy texture of polenta and the aromatic blend of herbs, it's a delicious twist on traditional pizza crusts.

Total Time: 1 hour

Servings: Makes one 12-inch pizza crust

Ingredients:
- 1 cup polenta (cornmeal)
- 3 cups water
- 1 tablespoon olive oil
- 1 teaspoon dried thyme
- 1 teaspoon dried rosemary
- 1/2 teaspoon garlic powder

- Salt and pepper to taste

Directions:

1. In a medium saucepan, bring the water to a boil. Gradually whisk in the polenta, stirring constantly to prevent lumps.
2. Reduce the heat to low and simmer, stirring frequently, for 20-25 minutes, or until the polenta is thick and creamy.
3. Remove the polenta from the heat and stir in the olive oil, dried thyme, dried rosemary, garlic powder, salt, and pepper.
4. Line a baking sheet with parchment paper. Pour the polenta mixture onto the prepared baking sheet and spread it out into a circle, about 1/4 inch thick.
5. Let the polenta crust cool and firm up for about 30 minutes.
6. Preheat your oven to 425°F (220°C). Bake the polenta crust in the preheated oven for 20-25 minutes, or until the edges are crispy and golden brown.

7. Remove from the oven and let cool slightly before adding your favorite toppings.
8. Return the pizza to the oven and bake for an additional 10-15 minutes, or until the toppings are heated through and the cheese is melted.
9. Slice and serve hot.

Nutritional Information (per serving):

- Calories: 160 kcal
- Fat: 3g
- Carbohydrates: 30g
- Fiber: 3g
- Protein: 4g

9. Chickpea Flour Gluten-Free Crust Pizza

Intro: This chickpea flour gluten-free crust pizza is perfect for those with gluten sensitivities or dietary restrictions. With the nutty flavor of chickpea flour and a crispy texture, it's a delicious alternative to traditional pizza crusts.

Total Time: 40 minutes

Low Fat Pizza Recipes

Servings: Makes one 12-inch pizza crust

Ingredients:
- 1 cup chickpea flour
- 1 cup water
- 1 tablespoon olive oil
- 1/2 teaspoon dried basil
- 1/2 teaspoon dried oregano
- 1/4 teaspoon garlic powder
- Salt and pepper to taste

Directions:
1. In a mixing bowl, whisk together the chickpea flour, water, olive oil, dried basil, dried oregano, garlic powder, salt, and pepper until smooth.
2. Let the batter rest for 10-15 minutes to allow the flavors to meld.
3. Preheat your oven to 425°F (220°C). Line a baking sheet with parchment paper.
4. Pour the batter onto the prepared baking sheet and spread it out into a circle, about 1/4 inch thick.
5. Bake in the preheated oven for 20-25 minutes, or until the crust is set and lightly golden brown.

6. Remove from the oven and let cool slightly before adding your favorite toppings.
7. Return the pizza to the oven and bake for an additional 10-15 minutes, or until the toppings are heated through and the cheese is melted.
8. Slice and serve hot.

Nutritional Information (per serving):
- Calories: 150 kcal
- Fat: 6g
- Carbohydrates: 18g
- Fiber: 5g
- Protein: 7g

10. Buckwheat and Sunflower Seed Crust Pizza

Intro: This buckwheat and sunflower seed crust pizza offers a hearty and nutritious base for your favorite toppings. With the earthy flavor of buckwheat and the crunch of sunflower seeds, it's a delightful twist on traditional pizza crusts.

Total Time: 50 minutes

Servings: Makes one 12-inch pizza crust

Ingredients:
- 1 cup buckwheat flour
- 1/4 cup sunflower seeds
- 1/2 teaspoon baking powder
- 1/4 teaspoon salt
- 1/2 cup water
- 1 tablespoon olive oil

Directions:
1. Preheat your oven to 400°F (200°C). Line a baking sheet with parchment paper.
2. In a food processor, pulse the sunflower seeds until finely ground.
3. In a large mixing bowl, combine the buckwheat flour, ground sunflower seeds, baking powder, and salt.
4. Stir in the water and olive oil until a dough forms.
5. Transfer the dough to the prepared baking sheet and spread it out into a circle, about 1/4 inch thick.

6. Bake in the preheated oven for 20-25 minutes, or until the crust is set and lightly golden brown.
7. Remove from the oven and let cool slightly before adding your favorite toppings.
8. Return the pizza to the oven and bake for an additional 10-15 minutes, or until the toppings are heated through and the cheese is melted.
9. Slice and serve hot.

Nutritional Information (per serving):
- Calories: 160 kcal
- Fat: 7g
- Carbohydrates: 20g
- Fiber: 4g
- Protein: 5g

Chapter 3: Low fat healthy sauce alternatives

1. Homemade Roasted Red Pepper Sauce

Intro: This homemade roasted red pepper sauce adds a burst of flavor to your pizza while keeping it light and healthy. Made with roasted red peppers, garlic, and herbs, it's a delicious alternative to traditional pizza sauces.

Total Time: 30 minutes

Servings: Makes about 1 cup of sauce

Ingredients:
- 2 large red bell peppers
- 2 cloves garlic, minced
- 1 tablespoon olive oil
- 1 tablespoon tomato paste
- 1 teaspoon dried oregano
- Salt and pepper to taste

Directions:

1. Preheat your broiler to high. Place the red bell peppers on a baking sheet and broil, turning occasionally, until charred and blistered on all sides, about 10-15 minutes.
2. Transfer the roasted peppers to a bowl and cover with plastic wrap. Let them steam for 10 minutes, then peel off the skins and remove the seeds.
3. In a blender or food processor, combine the roasted peppers, minced garlic, olive oil, tomato paste, dried oregano, salt, and pepper. Blend until smooth.
4. Taste and adjust the seasoning, if needed.
5. Use the sauce immediately on your pizza, or store it in an airtight container in the refrigerator for up to one week.

Nutritional Information (per serving - 2 tablespoons):

- Calories: 30 kcal
- Fat: 2g
- Carbohydrates: 3g
- Fiber: 1g

- Protein: 1g

2. Greek Yogurt Pesto Sauce

Intro: This Greek yogurt pesto sauce is a creamy and tangy alternative to traditional pesto, perfect for adding a burst of flavor to your pizza. Made with Greek yogurt, fresh basil, garlic, and Parmesan cheese, it's a lighter option without sacrificing taste.

Total Time: 10 minutes

Servings: Makes about 1 cup of sauce

Ingredients:
- 1 cup fresh basil leaves
- 1/4 cup grated Parmesan cheese
- 1/4 cup Greek yogurt
- 2 cloves garlic
- 2 tablespoons pine nuts or walnuts (optional)
- 2 tablespoons olive oil
- Salt and pepper to taste

Directions:

1. In a food processor, combine the basil leaves, Parmesan cheese, Greek yogurt, garlic, and pine nuts or walnuts (if using). Pulse until finely chopped.
2. With the food processor running, slowly drizzle in the olive oil until the mixture is smooth and well combined.
3. Season with salt and pepper to taste, and pulse a few more times to mix.
4. Use the sauce immediately on your pizza, or store it in an airtight container in the refrigerator for up to one week.

Nutritional Information (per serving - 2 tablespoons):

- Calories: 50 kcal
- Fat: 4g
- Carbohydrates: 1g
- Fiber: 0g
- Protein: 2g

3. Spicy Sriracha Marinara Sauce

Intro: This spicy Sriracha marinara sauce adds a kick to your pizza with its bold flavor and heat. Made with marinara sauce and Sriracha sauce, it's a simple yet delicious way to spice up your pizza without adding extra fat.

Total Time: 15 minutes

Servings: Makes about 1 cup of sauce

Ingredients:
- 1 cup marinara sauce (store-bought or homemade)
- 2 tablespoons Sriracha sauce (adjust to taste)
- 1 teaspoon olive oil (optional)
- 1/2 teaspoon dried basil
- 1/2 teaspoon dried oregano
- Salt and pepper to taste

Directions:
1. In a small saucepan, heat the olive oil over medium heat (if using).
2. Add the marinara sauce, Sriracha sauce, dried basil, dried oregano, salt, and pepper to the saucepan. Stir to combine.

3. Cook the sauce for 5-7 minutes, stirring occasionally, until heated through and slightly thickened.
4. Taste and adjust the seasoning or spiciness level as needed.
5. Use the sauce immediately on your pizza, or store it in an airtight container in the refrigerator for up to one week.

Nutritional Information (per serving - 2 tablespoons):
- Calories: 20 kcal
- Fat: 1g
- Carbohydrates: 3g
- Fiber: 1g
- Protein: 1g

4. Avocado Basil Sauce

Intro: This creamy avocado basil sauce adds richness and freshness to your pizza without the need for heavy cheeses or oils. With ripe avocados, fresh basil, and a hint of lemon juice, it's a flavorful and nutritious alternative to traditional pizza sauces.

Total Time: 10 minutes

Servings: Makes about 1 cup of sauce

Ingredients:
- 1 ripe avocado, peeled and pitted
- 1/2 cup fresh basil leaves
- 1 clove garlic, minced
- 2 tablespoons lemon juice
- Salt and pepper to taste
- Water, as needed

Directions:
1. In a food processor or blender, combine the ripe avocado, fresh basil leaves, minced garlic, lemon juice, salt, and pepper.
2. Blend until smooth, adding water as needed to reach your desired consistency.
3. Taste and adjust the seasoning, adding more salt, pepper, or lemon juice if desired.
4. Use the sauce immediately on your pizza, or store it in an airtight container

in the refrigerator for up to one day (note: avocado may brown over time).

Nutritional Information (per serving - 2 tablespoons):
- Calories: 40 kcal
- Fat: 3g
- Carbohydrates: 3g
- Fiber: 2g
- Protein: 1g

5. Lemon Garlic White Bean Sauce

Intro: This lemon garlic white bean sauce is creamy, flavorful, and packed with protein, making it a nutritious choice for pizza night. With white beans, garlic, lemon juice, and a touch of olive oil, it's a light and tangy alternative to traditional pizza sauces.

Total Time: 10 minutes

Servings: Makes about 1 cup of sauce

Ingredients:
- 1 can (15 ounces) white beans, drained and rinsed

- 2 cloves garlic, minced
- 2 tablespoons lemon juice
- 1 tablespoon olive oil
- Salt and pepper to taste
- Water, as needed

Directions:

1. In a food processor or blender, combine the white beans, minced garlic, lemon juice, olive oil, salt, and pepper.
2. Blend until smooth, adding water as needed to reach your desired consistency.
3. Taste and adjust the seasoning, adding more salt, pepper, or lemon juice if desired.
4. Use the sauce immediately on your pizza, or store it in an airtight container in the refrigerator for up to one day.

Nutritional Information (per serving - 2 tablespoons):

- Calories: 30 kcal
- Fat: 1g
- Carbohydrates: 5g
- Fiber: 1g
- Protein: 2g

6. Balsamic Glaze Drizzle

Intro: This balsamic glaze drizzle adds a sweet and tangy flavor to your pizza, elevating it to gourmet status. Made with balsamic vinegar and a touch of honey or sugar, it's a simple yet sophisticated sauce alternative that pairs well with a variety of toppings.

Total Time: 15 minutes

Servings: Makes about 1/2 cup of glaze

Ingredients:
- 1 cup balsamic vinegar
- 2 tablespoons honey or sugar

Directions:
1. In a small saucepan, combine the balsamic vinegar and honey or sugar.
2. Bring the mixture to a boil over medium-high heat, then reduce the heat to low and simmer for 10-12 minutes, or until the glaze has thickened and reduced by half. It should coat the back of a spoon.

3. Remove from heat and let the glaze cool slightly before using.
4. Drizzle the balsamic glaze over your cooked pizza just before serving, or serve it on the side for dipping.

Nutritional Information (per serving - 1 tablespoon):
- Calories: 40 kcal
- Fat: 0g
- Carbohydrates: 10g
- Fiber: 0g
- Protein: 0g

7. Chipotle Hummus Spread

Intro: This chipotle hummus spread adds a smoky and spicy kick to your pizza, along with a boost of protein and fiber. Made with chickpeas, tahini, chipotle peppers, and spices, it's a flavorful and satisfying sauce alternative that's sure to please your taste buds.

Total Time: 10 minutes

Servings: Makes about 1 cup of spread

Ingredients:
- 1 can (15 ounces) chickpeas, drained and rinsed
- 2 tablespoons tahini
- 2 chipotle peppers in adobo sauce
- 1 tablespoon lemon juice
- 1 clove garlic
- 1/2 teaspoon ground cumin
- 1/4 teaspoon smoked paprika
- Salt to taste
- Water, as needed

Directions:
1. In a food processor or blender, combine the chickpeas, tahini, chipotle peppers, lemon juice, garlic, ground cumin, smoked paprika, and salt.
2. Blend until smooth, adding water as needed to reach your desired consistency.
3. Taste and adjust the seasoning, adding more salt or chipotle peppers if desired.
4. Use the chipotle hummus spread immediately on your pizza, or store it in an airtight container in the refrigerator for up to one week.

Nutritional Information (per serving - 2 tablespoons):
- Calories: 50 kcal
- Fat: 2g
- Carbohydrates: 6g
- Fiber: 2g
- Protein: 2g

8. Walnut and Sun-Dried Tomato Pesto

Intro: This walnut and sun-dried tomato pesto is a rich and flavorful sauce alternative for your pizza. With the nuttiness of walnuts and the sweetness of sun-dried tomatoes, it adds depth of flavor to any pizza combination.

Total Time: 15 minutes

Servings: Makes about 1 cup of pesto

Ingredients:
- 1 cup fresh basil leaves
- 1/4 cup walnuts
- 1/4 cup sun-dried tomatoes (packed in oil), drained
- 1 clove garlic

- 2 tablespoons grated Parmesan cheese
- 2 tablespoons olive oil
- Salt and pepper to taste

Directions:
1. In a food processor, combine the fresh basil leaves, walnuts, sun-dried tomatoes, garlic, and Parmesan cheese.
2. Pulse until the ingredients are finely chopped.
3. With the food processor running, slowly drizzle in the olive oil until the pesto reaches your desired consistency.
4. Season with salt and pepper to taste, and pulse a few more times to mix.
5. Use the walnut and sun-dried tomato pesto immediately on your pizza, or store it in an airtight container in the refrigerator for up to one week.

Nutritional Information (per serving - 2 tablespoons):
- Calories: 80 kcal
- Fat: 7g
- Carbohydrates: 3g
- Fiber: 1g
- Protein: 2g

9. Cilantro Lime Yogurt Sauce

Intro: This cilantro lime yogurt sauce is bright, tangy, and refreshing, making it the perfect complement to your pizza. With Greek yogurt, fresh cilantro, lime juice, and a hint of garlic, it adds a burst of flavor without the extra calories.

Total Time: 10 minutes
Servings: Makes about 1 cup of sauce

Ingredients:
- 1 cup Greek yogurt
- 1/4 cup fresh cilantro leaves
- 2 tablespoons lime juice
- 1 clove garlic, minced
- Salt and pepper to taste

Directions:
1. In a blender or food processor, combine the Greek yogurt, cilantro leaves, lime juice, minced garlic, salt, and pepper.
2. Blend until the mixture is smooth and well combined.

3. Taste and adjust the seasoning, adding more salt, pepper, or lime juice if desired.
4. Use the cilantro lime yogurt sauce immediately on your pizza, or store it in an airtight container in the refrigerator for up to one week.

Nutritional Information (per serving - 2 tablespoons):
- Calories: 15 kcal
- Fat: 0g
- Carbohydrates: 2g
- Fiber: 0g
- Protein: 2g

10. Beet and Goat Cheese Spread

Intro: This beet and goat cheese spread adds a unique flavor and vibrant color to your pizza. Made with roasted beets, tangy goat cheese, and a touch of honey, it's a deliciously creamy and slightly sweet sauce alternative that's sure to impress.

Total Time: 45 minutes (including roasting time for beets)

Servings: Makes about 1 cup of spread

Ingredients:
- 2 medium beets, roasted, peeled, and diced
- 4 ounces goat cheese
- 1 tablespoon honey
- 1 tablespoon olive oil
- Salt and pepper to taste

Directions:
1. Preheat your oven to 400°F (200°C). Wrap the beets individually in aluminum foil and place them on a baking sheet. Roast for 30-40 minutes, or until the beets are tender when pierced with a fork. Let them cool, then peel and dice.
2. In a food processor, combine the roasted diced beets, goat cheese, honey, olive oil, salt, and pepper.
3. Pulse until the mixture is smooth and well combined.

4. Taste and adjust the seasoning, adding more salt, pepper, or honey if desired.

5. Use the beet and goat cheese spread immediately on your pizza, or store it in an airtight container in the refrigerator for up to one week.

Nutritional Information (per serving - 2 tablespoons):
- Calories: 60 kcal
- Fat: 4g
- Carbohydrates: 5g
- Fiber: 1g
- Protein: 2g

Chapter 4: Low-fat lean protein toppings

1. Grilled Chicken Breast

Intro: Grilled chicken breast is a classic and versatile topping for pizza, adding lean protein and savory flavor to your meal.

Total Time: 20 minutes

Servings: Depends on the amount of chicken used

Ingredients:
- Boneless, skinless chicken breasts
- Olive oil
- Salt and pepper
- Italian seasoning (optional)

Directions:
1. Preheat your grill to medium-high heat.
2. Season the chicken breasts with olive oil, salt, pepper, and Italian seasoning, if desired.
3. Grill the chicken for 6-8 minutes per side, or until cooked through and no longer pink in the center.
4. Let the chicken rest for a few minutes before slicing it thinly.
5. Top your pizza with the grilled chicken slices before baking or add them as a topping after baking.

Nutritional Information (per serving - 3 oz of cooked chicken breast):
- Calories: 120 kcal
- Fat: 2g
- Carbohydrates: 0g
- Protein: 26g

2. Turkey Pepperoni

Intro: Turkey pepperoni is a leaner alternative to traditional pork pepperoni, offering the same bold flavor with less fat.

Total Time: 10 minutes

Servings: Depends on the amount of pepperoni used

Ingredients:
- Turkey pepperoni slices

Directions:
1. Preheat your oven to 400°F (200°C).
2. Place the turkey pepperoni slices on a baking sheet lined with parchment paper.
3. Bake in the preheated oven for 5-7 minutes, or until the edges are crispy.
4. Remove from the oven and blot off any excess grease with paper towels.
5. Use the turkey pepperoni slices as a topping for your pizza before or after baking.

Nutritional Information (per serving - 15 slices):
- Calories: 70 kcal
- Fat: 4g
- Carbohydrates: 0g
- Protein: 8g

3. Shrimp

Intro: Shrimp adds a delightful seafood flavor and lean protein to your pizza, making it a refreshing and healthy option.

Total Time: 15 minutes
Servings: Depends on the amount of shrimp used

Ingredients:
- Shrimp, peeled and deveined
- Olive oil
- Salt and pepper
- Garlic powder (optional)
- Lemon zest (optional)
- Red pepper flakes (optional)

Directions:

1. In a bowl, toss the shrimp with olive oil, salt, pepper, and any optional seasonings like garlic powder, lemon zest, or red pepper flakes.
2. Heat a skillet over medium-high heat and add the seasoned shrimp.
3. Cook the shrimp for 2-3 minutes per side, or until they turn pink and opaque.
4. Remove the shrimp from the skillet and let them cool slightly.
5. Arrange the cooked shrimp as a topping on your pizza before or after baking.

Nutritional Information (per serving - 3 oz of cooked shrimp):
- Calories: 90 kcal
- Fat: 1g
- Carbohydrates: 0g
- Protein: 20g

4. Lean Ground Turkey

Intro: Lean ground turkey is a versatile and healthy protein option for pizza, providing a satisfying meaty texture without excess fat.

Total Time: 20 minutes

Servings: Depends on the amount of ground turkey used

Ingredients:
- Lean ground turkey
- Olive oil
- Salt and pepper
- Onion powder (optional)
- Garlic powder (optional)
- Italian seasoning (optional)

Directions:
1. Heat a skillet over medium heat and add a drizzle of olive oil.
2. Add the lean ground turkey to the skillet, breaking it apart with a spoon.
3. Season the turkey with salt, pepper, and any optional seasonings like onion powder, garlic powder, or Italian seasoning.
4. Cook the ground turkey for 8-10 minutes, stirring occasionally, until it is browned and cooked through.

5. Drain any excess fat from the skillet and let the ground turkey cool slightly.
6. Spread the cooked ground turkey evenly over your pizza crust before adding other toppings or bake it along with the pizza.

Nutritional Information (per serving - 3 oz of cooked ground turkey):
- Calories: 120 kcal
- Fat: 5g
- Carbohydrates: 0g
- Protein: 20g

5. Tofu Cubes

Intro: Tofu cubes are a plant-based protein option that adds a creamy texture and subtle flavor to your pizza, making it suitable for vegetarians and vegans.

Total Time: 30 minutes

Servings: Depends on the amount of tofu used

Ingredients:
- Firm tofu, pressed and cubed
- Olive oil
- Soy sauce or tamari
- Garlic powder
- Onion powder
- Paprika
- Salt and pepper

Directions:
1. Preheat your oven to 400°F (200°C) and line a baking sheet with parchment paper.
2. In a bowl, toss the tofu cubes with olive oil, soy sauce or tamari, garlic powder, onion powder, paprika, salt, and pepper, ensuring the tofu is evenly coated.
3. Spread the tofu cubes in a single layer on the prepared baking sheet.
4. Bake for 20-25 minutes, flipping halfway through, until the tofu is golden and crispy on the outside.
5. Remove from the oven and let the tofu cool slightly before using it as a pizza topping.

Nutritional Information (per serving - 3 oz of cooked tofu):
- Calories: 70 kcal
- Fat: 4g
- Carbohydrates: 2g
- Protein: 8g

6. Turkey Sausage Crumbles

Intro: Turkey sausage crumbles offer a flavorful and lean alternative to traditional pork sausage, making them a healthier option for topping your pizza.

Total Time: 15 minutes

Servings: Depends on the amount of turkey sausage used

Ingredients:
- Turkey sausage, casings removed
- Olive oil
- Italian seasoning
- Garlic powder
- Onion powder
- Salt and pepper

Directions:

1. Heat a skillet over medium heat and add a drizzle of olive oil.
2. Add the turkey sausage to the skillet, breaking it apart into crumbles with a spoon.
3. Season the turkey sausage with Italian seasoning, garlic powder, onion powder, salt, and pepper.
4. Cook the turkey sausage crumbles for 8-10 minutes, stirring occasionally, until they are browned and cooked through.
5. Remove any excess fat from the skillet and let the turkey sausage crumbles cool slightly before using them as a pizza topping.

Nutritional Information (per serving - 3 oz of cooked turkey sausage):
- Calories: 120 kcal
- Fat: 6g
- Carbohydrates: 2g
- Protein: 14g

7. Grilled Tofu Strips

Intro: Grilled tofu strips are a delicious and nutritious topping option for pizza, providing a meaty texture and a subtle flavor that pairs well with a variety of other ingredients.

Total Time: 30 minutes (including marinating time)

Servings: Depends on the amount of tofu used

Ingredients:
- Firm tofu, pressed and sliced into strips
- Soy sauce or tamari
- Rice vinegar
- Sesame oil
- Garlic powder
- Ginger powder
- Salt and pepper

Directions:
1. In a bowl, whisk together soy sauce or tamari, rice vinegar, sesame oil, garlic powder, ginger powder, salt, and pepper to make the marinade.
2. Place the tofu strips in a shallow dish and pour the marinade over them, ensuring they are well coated. Let them

marinate for at least 20 minutes, or longer for a stronger flavor.

3. Preheat a grill or grill pan over medium-high heat. Remove the tofu strips from the marinade and grill them for 2-3 minutes per side, or until they are lightly charred and heated through.

4. Remove from the grill and let the tofu cool slightly before using it as a pizza topping.

Nutritional Information (per serving - 3 oz of grilled tofu strips):
- Calories: 80 kcal
- Fat: 4g
- Carbohydrates: 3g
- Protein: 9g

8. White Beans

Intro: White beans are a versatile and protein-rich topping for pizza, offering a creamy texture and mild flavor that complements a variety of other ingredients.

Total Time: 10 minutes

Servings: Depends on the amount of white beans used

Ingredients:
- Canned white beans, drained and rinsed
- Olive oil
- Garlic powder
- Onion powder
- Italian seasoning
- Salt and pepper

Directions:
1. Heat a skillet over medium heat and add a drizzle of olive oil.
2. Add the white beans to the skillet and season with garlic powder, onion powder, Italian seasoning, salt, and pepper.
3. Cook the white beans for 5-7 minutes, stirring occasionally, until they are heated through and slightly golden.
4. Remove from the heat and let the white beans cool slightly before using them as a pizza topping.

Nutritional Information (per serving - 1/2 cup of cooked white beans):
- Calories: 100 kcal
- Fat: 0g
- Carbohydrates: 20g
- Protein: 7g

9. Cottage Cheese

Intro: Cottage cheese is a creamy and low-fat protein option for pizza, adding a rich texture and mild flavor that pairs well with a variety of toppings.

Total Time: 5 minutes

Servings: Depends on the amount of cottage cheese used

Ingredients:
- Cottage cheese

Directions:
1. Simply spoon cottage cheese onto your pizza crust as a topping before or after baking.

2. Spread the cottage cheese evenly over the crust, or dollop it in small amounts over other toppings.

Nutritional Information (per serving - 1/2 cup of cottage cheese):
- Calories: 90 kcal
- Fat: 2g
- Carbohydrates: 3g
- Protein: 14g

10. Egg Whites

Intro: Egg whites are a high-protein, low-fat topping option for pizza, adding a fluffy texture and subtle flavor to your dish.

Total Time: 10 minutes

Servings: Depends on the amount of egg whites used

Ingredients:
- Egg whites
- Salt and pepper
- Cooking spray or olive oil (for cooking)

Directions:
1. In a bowl, whisk together the egg whites with a pinch of salt and pepper.
2. Heat a non-stick skillet over medium heat and lightly coat it with cooking spray or olive oil.
3. Pour the egg whites into the skillet, spreading them out into an even layer.
4. Cook the egg whites for 2-3 minutes, or until they are set on the bottom and beginning to set on top.
5. Carefully flip the egg whites and cook for an additional 1-2 minutes, or until fully cooked through.
6. Remove from the skillet and let the cooked egg whites cool slightly before using them as a pizza topping.

Nutritional Information (per serving - 3 egg whites):
- Calories: 50 kcal
- Fat: 0g
- Carbohydrates: 1g
- Protein: 11g

Enjoy experimenting with these low-fat lean protein toppings to create delicious and nutritious pizzas at home!

Chapter 5: Abundant veggie creations

1. Garden Veggie Delight

Intro: Garden Veggie Delight pizza is a celebration of fresh, colorful vegetables atop a crispy crust, making it a flavorful and nutritious meal.

Low Fat Pizza Recipes

Total Time: 30 minutes

Servings: 4

Ingredients:
- 1 pre-made whole wheat pizza crust
- 1/2 cup tomato sauce
- 1 cup sliced bell peppers (red, green, and yellow)
- 1 cup sliced mushrooms
- 1 cup sliced zucchini
- 1/2 cup sliced red onion
- 1 cup cherry tomatoes, halved
- 1 cup spinach leaves
- 1/2 cup shredded part-skim mozzarella cheese
- 1 tablespoon olive oil
- Salt and pepper to taste
- Italian seasoning (optional)

Directions:
1. Preheat your oven to 425°F (220°C).
2. Place the pizza crust on a baking sheet lined with parchment paper.
3. Spread the tomato sauce evenly over the crust, leaving a small border around the edges.

4. Arrange the sliced vegetables over the sauce, layering them evenly.
5. Drizzle the olive oil over the vegetables and season with salt, pepper, and Italian seasoning if desired.
6. Sprinkle the shredded mozzarella cheese over the top of the vegetables.
7. Bake the pizza in the preheated oven for 15-20 minutes, or until the crust is golden and the cheese is melted and bubbly.
8. Remove from the oven and let the pizza cool for a few minutes before slicing and serving.

Nutritional Information (per serving):
- Calories: 250 kcal
- Fat: 8g
- Carbohydrates: 35g
- Fiber: 5g
- Protein: 10g

2. Mediterranean Veggie Feast

Intro: Mediterranean Veggie Feast pizza brings the flavors of the Mediterranean to your table with a colorful array of veggies, olives, and feta cheese.

Total Time: 35 minutes

Servings: 4

Ingredients:
- 1 pre-made whole wheat pizza crust
- 1/2 cup hummus
- 1 cup chopped roasted red peppers
- 1 cup sliced black olives
- 1/2 cup sliced red onion
- 1/2 cup crumbled feta cheese
- 1/4 cup chopped fresh parsley
- 1 tablespoon olive oil
- Salt and pepper to taste
- Lemon wedges (for serving)

Directions:
1. Preheat your oven to 425°F (220°C).
2. Spread the hummus evenly over the pizza crust.
3. Arrange the roasted red peppers, black olives, and red onion slices on top of the hummus.
4. Sprinkle the crumbled feta cheese and chopped parsley over the vegetables.

5. Drizzle the olive oil over the pizza and season with salt and pepper.
6. Bake the pizza in the preheated oven for 15-20 minutes, or until the crust is crisp and the toppings are heated through.
7. Remove from the oven and let the pizza cool slightly before slicing.
8. Serve with lemon wedges for squeezing over the pizza, if desired.

Nutritional Information (per serving):
- Calories: 280 kcal
- Fat: 12g
- Carbohydrates: 32g
- Fiber: 6g
- Protein: 10g

3. Roasted Veggie Extravaganza

Intro: Roasted Veggie Extravaganza pizza is bursting with flavor from an assortment of roasted vegetables, creating a hearty and satisfying meal.

Total Time: 40 minutes

Servings: 4

Ingredients:
- 1 pre-made whole wheat pizza crust
- 1 cup cherry tomatoes, halved
- 1 cup diced eggplant
- 1 cup diced zucchini
- 1 cup sliced bell peppers (red, green, and yellow)
- 1/2 cup sliced red onion
- 2 cloves garlic, minced
- 2 tablespoons balsamic vinegar
- 1 tablespoon olive oil
- Salt and pepper to taste
- Fresh basil leaves for garnish

Directions:
1. Preheat your oven to 425°F (220°C).
2. In a large bowl, toss the cherry tomatoes, diced eggplant, diced zucchini, sliced bell peppers, sliced red onion, and minced garlic with balsamic vinegar, olive oil, salt, and pepper.
3. Spread the vegetable mixture evenly on a baking sheet lined with parchment paper.

4. Roast the vegetables in the preheated oven for 20-25 minutes, or until they are tender and slightly caramelized.
5. Remove from the oven and set aside.
6. Place the pizza crust on a separate baking sheet.
7. Spread the roasted vegetables over the pizza crust.
8. Return the pizza to the oven and bake for an additional 10 minutes, or until the crust is crisp.
9. Remove from the oven, garnish with fresh basil leaves, and serve hot.

Nutritional Information (per serving):
- Calories: 230 kcal
- Fat: 6g
- Carbohydrates: 38g
- Fiber: 7g
- Protein: 7g

4. Spinach and Artichoke Delight

Intro: Spinach and Artichoke Delight pizza combines the creamy goodness of spinach and artichoke dip with the crunch of a pizza crust for a delicious and healthy twist on a classic appetizer.

Total Time: 25 minutes

Servings: 4

Ingredients:
- 1 pre-made whole wheat pizza crust
- 1 cup fresh spinach leaves
- 1 cup canned artichoke hearts, chopped
- 1/2 cup low-fat cream cheese
- 1/4 cup plain Greek yogurt
- 1/4 cup grated Parmesan cheese
- 2 cloves garlic, minced
- 1 tablespoon lemon juice
- Salt and pepper to taste
- Red pepper flakes (optional)

Directions:
1. Preheat your oven to 425°F (220°C).
2. In a mixing bowl, combine the low-fat cream cheese, Greek yogurt, grated Parmesan cheese, minced garlic, lemon juice, salt, and pepper.

3. Spread the cream cheese mixture evenly over the pizza crust.
4. Arrange the fresh spinach leaves and chopped artichoke hearts on top of the cream cheese mixture.
5. If desired, sprinkle with red pepper flakes for extra heat.
6. Bake the pizza in the preheated oven for 12-15 minutes, or until the crust is golden and the toppings are heated through.
7. Remove from the oven and let the pizza cool for a few minutes before slicing and serving.

Nutritional Information (per serving):
- Calories: 250 kcal
- Fat: 9g
- Carbohydrates: 30g
- Fiber: 6g

5. Grilled Veggie Paradise

Intro: Grilled Veggie Paradise pizza features a smoky blend of grilled vegetables atop a crispy crust, offering a burst of flavor in every bite.

Total Time: 30 minutes

Servings: 4

Ingredients:
- 1 pre-made whole wheat pizza crust
- 1 cup sliced zucchini
- 1 cup sliced bell peppers (red, green, and yellow)
- 1 cup sliced eggplant
- 1 cup sliced red onion
- 1/4 cup balsamic vinegar
- 2 tablespoons olive oil
- Salt and pepper to taste
- Fresh basil leaves for garnish

Directions:
1. Preheat your grill to medium-high heat.
2. In a large bowl, toss the sliced zucchini, bell peppers, eggplant, and red onion with balsamic vinegar, olive oil, salt, and pepper.
3. Place the vegetables on the preheated grill and cook for 8-10 minutes, turning occasionally, until they are tender and lightly charred.

4. Remove the grilled vegetables from the grill and set aside.
5. Place the pizza crust on the grill and cook for 2-3 minutes on each side, until lightly toasted.
6. Remove the crust from the grill and place it on a baking sheet.
7. Arrange the grilled vegetables on top of the crust.
8. Return the pizza to the grill and cook for an additional 5-7 minutes, or until the crust is crisp and the toppings are heated through.
9. Remove from the grill, garnish with fresh basil leaves, and serve hot.

Nutritional Information (per serving):
- Calories: 260 kcal
- Fat: 9g
- Carbohydrates: 38g
- Fiber: 7g
- Protein: 8g

6. Veggie Pesto Delight

Intro: Veggie Pesto Delight pizza combines the vibrant flavors of homemade pesto sauce with an assortment of fresh vegetables, creating a delicious and satisfying meal.

Total Time: 25 minutes

Servings: 4

Ingredients:
- 1 pre-made whole wheat pizza crust
- 1/2 cup homemade or store-bought pesto sauce
- 1 cup cherry tomatoes, halved
- 1 cup sliced bell peppers (red, green, and yellow)
- 1 cup sliced mushrooms
- 1/2 cup sliced red onion
- 1/4 cup pine nuts (optional)
- Salt and pepper to taste
- Fresh basil leaves for garnish

Directions:
1. Preheat your oven to 425°F (220°C).
2. Spread the pesto sauce evenly over the pizza crust.
3. Arrange the cherry tomatoes, sliced bell peppers, mushrooms, and red onion on top of the pesto sauce.

4. If desired, sprinkle pine nuts over the vegetables for added crunch.
5. Season with salt and pepper to taste.
6. Bake the pizza in the preheated oven for 12-15 minutes, or until the crust is golden and the toppings are heated through.
7. Remove from the oven and let the pizza cool for a few minutes before slicing.
8. Garnish with fresh basil leaves before serving.

Nutritional Information (per serving):
- Calories: 290 kcal
- Fat: 15g
- Carbohydrates: 30g
- Fiber: 6g
- Protein: 8g

7. Summer Veggie Harvest

Intro: Summer Veggie Harvest pizza captures the essence of the season with a medley of fresh summer vegetables, creating a colorful and flavorful dish that's perfect for warm weather dining.

Low Fat Pizza Recipes

Total Time: 30 minutes

Servings: 4

Ingredients:
- 1 pre-made whole wheat pizza crust
- 1 cup diced tomatoes
- 1 cup sliced yellow squash
- 1 cup sliced zucchini
- 1 cup sliced bell peppers (red, green, and yellow)
- 1/2 cup sliced red onion
- 2 cloves garlic, minced
- 2 tablespoons olive oil
- Salt and pepper to taste
- Fresh basil leaves for garnish

Directions:
1. Preheat your oven to 425°F (220°C).
2. In a large bowl, toss the diced tomatoes, sliced yellow squash, sliced zucchini, sliced bell peppers, sliced red onion, and minced garlic with olive oil, salt, and pepper.
3. Spread the vegetable mixture evenly over the pizza crust.

4. Bake the pizza in the preheated oven for 15-20 minutes, or until the crust is golden and the vegetables are tender.
5. Remove from the oven and let the pizza cool for a few minutes before slicing.
6. Garnish with fresh basil leaves before serving.

Nutritional Information (per serving):
- Calories: 270 kcal
- Fat: 10g
- Carbohydrates: 38g
- Fiber: 7g
- Protein: 8g

8. Mushroom Madness

Intro: Mushroom Madness pizza is a savory delight featuring an abundance of mushrooms atop a crispy crust, creating a satisfying and flavorful dish for mushroom lovers.

Total Time: 25 minutes

Servings: 4
Ingredients:
- 1 pre-made whole wheat pizza crust

- 2 cups sliced mushrooms (such as button mushrooms, cremini mushrooms, or shiitake mushrooms)
- 1 cup sliced red onion
- 2 cloves garlic, minced
- 1 tablespoon olive oil
- Salt and pepper to taste
- Fresh thyme leaves for garnish (optional)

Directions:

1. Preheat your oven to 425°F (220°C).
2. In a skillet, heat the olive oil over medium heat. Add the sliced mushrooms, sliced red onion, and minced garlic.
3. Sauté the mushrooms, onion, and garlic for 5-7 minutes, or until the mushrooms are golden brown and the onions are caramelized. Season with salt and pepper to taste.
4. Spread the mushroom mixture evenly over the pizza crust.
5. Bake the pizza in the preheated oven for 12-15 minutes, or until the crust is golden and the toppings are heated through.

6. Remove from the oven and let the pizza cool for a few minutes before slicing.
7. Garnish with fresh thyme leaves before serving, if desired.

Nutritional Information (per serving):
- Calories: 240 kcal
- Fat: 8g
- Carbohydrates: 35g
- Fiber: 6g
- Protein: 8g

9. Zucchini Ribbon Delight

Intro: Zucchini Ribbon Delight pizza features delicate zucchini ribbons atop a crispy crust, offering a fresh and light option that's perfect for summer.

Total Time: 30 minutes

Servings: 4

Ingredients:
- 1 pre-made whole wheat pizza crust
- 2 medium zucchinis, washed and thinly sliced lengthwise into ribbons

- 1 cup cherry tomatoes, halved
- 1/2 cup crumbled feta cheese
- 2 tablespoons chopped fresh basil
- 1 tablespoon olive oil
- 1 tablespoon balsamic glaze (optional)
- Salt and pepper to taste

Directions:

1. Preheat your oven to 425°F (220°C).
2. Place the zucchini ribbons in a bowl and toss with olive oil, salt, and pepper until evenly coated.
3. Spread the zucchini ribbons evenly over the pizza crust.
4. Arrange the cherry tomatoes on top of the zucchini ribbons.
5. Sprinkle the crumbled feta cheese over the vegetables.
6. Bake the pizza in the preheated oven for 15-20 minutes, or until the crust is golden and the toppings are heated through.
7. Remove from the oven and let the pizza cool for a few minutes before slicing.
8. Garnish with chopped fresh basil and drizzle with balsamic glaze, if desired, before serving.

Nutritional Information (per serving):
- Calories: 280 kcal
- Fat: 11g
- Carbohydrates: 35g
- Fiber: 6g
- Protein: 10g

10. Garden Fresh Margherita

Intro: Garden Fresh Margherita pizza is a classic favorite featuring ripe tomatoes, fresh basil, and creamy mozzarella cheese on a crispy crust, offering a taste of Italy in every bite.

Total Time: 20 minutes

Servings: 4

Ingredients:
- 1 pre-made whole wheat pizza crust
- 1 cup sliced ripe tomatoes
- 1 cup fresh basil leaves
- 8 ounces fresh mozzarella cheese, thinly sliced
- 2 cloves garlic, minced

- 2 tablespoons olive oil
- Salt and pepper to taste

Directions:
1. Preheat your oven to 425°F (220°C).
2. Spread the minced garlic evenly over the pizza crust.
3. Arrange the sliced tomatoes on top of the garlic.
4. Place the fresh basil leaves on top of the tomatoes.
5. Arrange the slices of fresh mozzarella cheese over the basil leaves.
6. Drizzle the olive oil over the toppings and season with salt and pepper to taste.
7. Bake the pizza in the preheated oven for 12-15 minutes, or until the crust is golden and the cheese is melted and bubbly.
8. Remove from the oven and let the pizza cool for a few minutes before slicing and serving.

Nutritional Information (per serving):
- Calories: 320 kcal
- Fat: 15g
- Carbohydrates: 30g

- Fiber: 6g
- Protein: 15g

Chapter 6: Low-fat cheese selections

1. Lightened-Up Margherita

Intro: Lightened-Up Margherita pizza offers a healthier twist on the classic Italian favorite, featuring fresh tomatoes, basil, and reduced-fat mozzarella cheese on a crispy crust.

Total Time: 25 minutes

Servings: 4

Ingredients:
- 1 pre-made whole wheat pizza crust
- 1 cup sliced ripe tomatoes
- 1 cup fresh basil leaves
- 8 ounces reduced-fat mozzarella cheese, thinly sliced
- 2 cloves garlic, minced
- 2 tablespoons olive oil
- Salt and pepper to taste

Directions:
1. Preheat your oven to 425°F (220°C).

2. Spread the minced garlic evenly over the pizza crust.
3. Arrange the sliced tomatoes on top of the garlic.
4. Place the fresh basil leaves on top of the tomatoes.
5. Arrange the slices of reduced-fat mozzarella cheese over the basil leaves.
6. Drizzle the olive oil over the toppings and season with salt and pepper to taste.
7. Bake the pizza in the preheated oven for 12-15 minutes, or until the crust is golden and the cheese is melted and bubbly.
8. Remove from the oven and let the pizza cool for a few minutes before slicing and serving.

Nutritional Information (per serving):
- Calories: 250 kcal
- Fat: 9g
- Carbohydrates: 30g
- Fiber: 6g
- Protein: 12g

2. Skinny Veggie Supreme

Intro: Skinny Veggie Supreme pizza is loaded with colorful vegetables and topped with a blend of reduced-fat cheeses, offering a guilt-free indulgence packed with flavor and nutrition.

Total Time: 30 minutes

Servings: 4

Ingredients:
- 1 pre-made whole wheat pizza crust
- 1/2 cup tomato sauce
- 1 cup sliced bell peppers (red, green, and yellow)
- 1 cup sliced mushrooms
- 1/2 cup sliced red onion
- 1/2 cup sliced black olives
- 1 cup reduced-fat shredded mozzarella cheese
- 1/4 cup reduced-fat shredded cheddar cheese
- 1 tablespoon olive oil
- Salt and pepper to taste
- Italian seasoning (optional)

Directions:
1. Preheat your oven to 425°F (220°C).
2. Spread the tomato sauce evenly over the pizza crust.
3. Arrange the sliced bell peppers, mushrooms, red onion, and black olives on top of the sauce.
4. In a small bowl, mix together the reduced-fat shredded mozzarella and cheddar cheeses.
5. Sprinkle the cheese mixture over the vegetables.
6. Drizzle the olive oil over the toppings and season with salt, pepper, and Italian seasoning if desired.
7. Bake the pizza in the preheated oven for 15-20 minutes, or until the crust is golden and the cheese is melted and bubbly.
8. Remove from the oven and let the pizza cool for a few minutes before slicing and serving.

Nutritional Information (per serving):
- Calories: 280 kcal
- Fat: 10g
- Carbohydrates: 35g

- Fiber: 6g
- Protein: 14g

3. Lean and Green Pesto

Intro: Lean and Green Pesto pizza combines the vibrant flavors of homemade pesto sauce with a variety of fresh vegetables and reduced-fat cheese, creating a lighter and healthier version of a classic favorite.

Total Time: 25 minutes

Servings: 4

Ingredients:
- 1 pre-made whole wheat pizza crust
- 1/2 cup homemade or store-bought pesto sauce
- 1 cup cherry tomatoes, halved
- 1 cup sliced bell peppers (red, green, and yellow)
- 1 cup sliced mushrooms
- 1/2 cup sliced red onion
- 1/4 cup reduced-fat shredded mozzarella cheese

- 1/4 cup reduced-fat shredded Parmesan cheese
- 1 tablespoon olive oil
- Salt and pepper to taste

Directions:

1. Preheat your oven to 425°F (220°C).
2. Spread the pesto sauce evenly over the pizza crust.
3. Arrange the cherry tomatoes, sliced bell peppers, mushrooms, and red onion on top of the pesto sauce.
4. Sprinkle the reduced-fat shredded mozzarella and Parmesan cheeses over the vegetables.
5. Drizzle the olive oil over the toppings and season with salt and pepper to taste.
6. Bake the pizza in the preheated oven for 12-15 minutes, or until the crust is golden and the cheese is melted and bubbly.
7. Remove from the oven and let the pizza cool for a few minutes before slicing and serving.

Nutritional Information (per serving):
- Calories: 290 kcal

- Fat: 12g
- Carbohydrates: 30g
- Fiber: 6g
- Protein: 10g

4. Reduced-Fat Mediterranean Delight

Intro: Reduced-Fat Mediterranean Delight pizza showcases the flavors of the Mediterranean with a blend of sun-dried tomatoes, olives, and reduced-fat feta cheese on a crispy crust, offering a lighter take on a classic favorite.

Total Time: 30 minutes

Servings: 4

Ingredients:
- 1 pre-made whole wheat pizza crust
- 1/2 cup tomato sauce
- 1/4 cup chopped sun-dried tomatoes
- 1/4 cup sliced black olives
- 1/4 cup sliced Kalamata olives

- 1/2 cup reduced-fat crumbled feta cheese
- 1 tablespoon olive oil
- Salt and pepper to taste
- Fresh oregano leaves for garnish (optional)

Directions:

1. Preheat your oven to 425°F (220°C).
2. Spread the tomato sauce evenly over the pizza crust.
3. Scatter the chopped sun-dried tomatoes, sliced black olives, and sliced Kalamata olives over the sauce.
4. Sprinkle the reduced-fat crumbled feta cheese over the toppings.
5. Drizzle the olive oil over the pizza and season with salt and pepper to taste.
6. Bake the pizza in the preheated oven for 12-15 minutes, or until the crust is golden and the cheese is melted and bubbly.
7. Remove from the oven and let the pizza cool for a few minutes before slicing.
8. Garnish with fresh oregano leaves before serving, if desired.

Nutritional Information (per serving):
- Calories: 270 kcal
- Fat: 10g
- Carbohydrates: 35g
- Fiber: 6g
- Protein: 12g

5. Fresh Tomato and Ricotta

Intro: Fresh Tomato and Ricotta pizza features juicy slices of ripe tomatoes and creamy reduced-fat ricotta cheese on a crispy crust, offering a light and satisfying option for pizza lovers.

Total Time: 25 minutes

Servings: 4

Ingredients:
- 1 pre-made whole wheat pizza crust
- 1 cup sliced ripe tomatoes
- 1/2 cup reduced-fat ricotta cheese
- 2 tablespoons grated Parmesan cheese

- 2 cloves garlic, minced
- 1 tablespoon olive oil
- Salt and pepper to taste
- Fresh basil leaves for garnish

Directions:

1. Preheat your oven to 425°F (220°C).
2. Spread the minced garlic evenly over the pizza crust.
3. Arrange the sliced tomatoes on top of the garlic.
4. Dollop the reduced-fat ricotta cheese over the tomatoes.
5. Sprinkle the grated Parmesan cheese over the toppings.
6. Drizzle the olive oil over the pizza and season with salt and pepper to taste.
7. Bake the pizza in the preheated oven for 12-15 minutes, or until the crust is golden and the cheese is melted and bubbly.
8. Remove from the oven and let the pizza cool for a few minutes before slicing.
9. Garnish with fresh basil leaves before serving.

Nutritional Information (per serving):

- Calories: 240 kcal
- Fat: 9g
- Carbohydrates: 30g
- Fiber: 6g
- Protein: 10g

6. Garden Harvest with Reduced-Fat Mozzarella

Intro: Garden Harvest with Reduced-Fat Mozzarella pizza is packed with an assortment of fresh garden vegetables and topped with reduced-fat mozzarella cheese on a wholesome crust, creating a nutritious and flavorful meal.

Total Time: 30 minutes

Servings: 4

Ingredients:
- 1 pre-made whole wheat pizza crust
- 1/2 cup tomato sauce
- 1 cup sliced bell peppers (red, green, and yellow)
- 1 cup sliced mushrooms
- 1/2 cup sliced red onion

- 1/2 cup sliced black olives
- 1 cup reduced-fat shredded mozzarella cheese
- 1 tablespoon olive oil
- Salt and pepper to taste
- Italian seasoning (optional)

Directions:

1. Preheat your oven to 425°F (220°C).
2. Spread the tomato sauce evenly over the pizza crust.
3. Arrange the sliced bell peppers, mushrooms, red onion, and black olives on top of the sauce.
4. Sprinkle the reduced-fat shredded mozzarella cheese over the vegetables.
5. Drizzle the olive oil over the toppings and season with salt, pepper, and Italian seasoning if desired.
6. Bake the pizza in the preheated oven for 15-20 minutes, or until the crust is golden and the cheese is melted and bubbly.
7. Remove from the oven and let the pizza cool for a few minutes before slicing and serving.

Nutritional Information (per serving):
- Calories: 270 kcal
- Fat: 10g
- Carbohydrates: 35g
- Fiber: 6g
- Protein: 14g

7. Spinach and Feta Delight

Intro: Spinach and Feta Delight pizza is a flavorful combination of sautéed spinach, tangy reduced-fat feta cheese, and a hint of garlic on a crispy crust, offering a delicious and nutritious meal option.

Total Time: 25 minutes

Servings: 4

Ingredients:
- 1 pre-made whole wheat pizza crust
- 2 cups fresh spinach leaves
- 1/2 cup reduced-fat crumbled feta cheese
- 2 cloves garlic, minced
- 1 tablespoon olive oil
- Salt and pepper to taste

- Crushed red pepper flakes (optional)

Directions:
1. Preheat your oven to 425°F (220°C).
2. In a skillet, heat the olive oil over medium heat. Add the minced garlic and sauté for 1-2 minutes, until fragrant.
3. Add the fresh spinach leaves to the skillet and cook until wilted, about 2-3 minutes. Season with salt, pepper, and crushed red pepper flakes if desired.
4. Spread the sautéed spinach evenly over the pizza crust.
5. Sprinkle the reduced-fat crumbled feta cheese over the spinach.
6. Bake the pizza in the preheated oven for 12-15 minutes, or until the crust is golden and the cheese is melted and bubbly.
7. Remove from the oven and let the pizza cool for a few minutes before slicing and serving.

Nutritional Information (per serving):
- Calories: 230 kcal
- Fat: 9g
- Carbohydrates: 30g

- Fiber: 6g
- Protein: 10g

8. Skinny BBQ Chicken

Intro: Skinny BBQ Chicken pizza is a tasty combination of tender chicken, tangy barbecue sauce, and reduced-fat cheese on a crispy crust, offering a lighter alternative to traditional BBQ chicken pizza.

Total Time: 30 minutes
Servings: 4

Ingredients:
- 1 pre-made whole wheat pizza crust
- 1/2 cup barbecue sauce (low-sugar, if available)
- 1 cup cooked chicken breast, shredded
- 1/2 cup sliced red onion
- 1 cup reduced-fat shredded mozzarella cheese
- 1 tablespoon chopped fresh cilantro (optional)
- Olive oil cooking spray

Directions:

1. Preheat your oven to 425°F (220°C).
2. Spray a baking sheet with olive oil cooking spray and place the pizza crust on it.
3. Spread the barbecue sauce evenly over the pizza crust.
4. Sprinkle the shredded chicken evenly over the barbecue sauce.
5. Scatter the sliced red onion over the chicken.
6. Sprinkle the reduced-fat shredded mozzarella cheese over the toppings.
7. Bake the pizza in the preheated oven for 12-15 minutes, or until the crust is golden and the cheese is melted and bubbly.
8. Remove from the oven and let the pizza cool for a few minutes before slicing.
9. Garnish with chopped fresh cilantro, if desired, before serving.

Nutritional Information (per serving):
- Calories: 270 kcal
- Fat: 8g
- Carbohydrates: 35g
- Fiber: 6g
- Protein: 18g

9. Greek Yogurt Ranch Veggie

Intro: Greek Yogurt Ranch Veggie pizza is a creamy and flavorful option that combines the tangy taste of ranch dressing with fresh vegetables and reduced-fat cheese on a whole wheat crust, offering a guilt-free indulgence.

Total Time: 25 minutes

Servings: 4

Ingredients:
- 1 pre-made whole wheat pizza crust
- 1/2 cup plain Greek yogurt
- 2 tablespoons ranch seasoning mix
- 1 cup sliced cherry tomatoes
- 1 cup sliced cucumbers
- 1/2 cup sliced red onion
- 1 cup reduced-fat shredded mozzarella cheese
- Salt and pepper to taste

Directions:
1. Preheat your oven to 425°F (220°C).

2. In a small bowl, mix together the plain Greek yogurt and ranch seasoning mix until well combined.
3. Spread the Greek yogurt ranch mixture evenly over the pizza crust.
4. Arrange the sliced cherry tomatoes, cucumbers, and red onion on top of the ranch dressing.
5. Sprinkle the reduced-fat shredded mozzarella cheese over the vegetables.
6. Season with salt and pepper to taste.
7. Bake the pizza in the preheated oven for 12-15 minutes, or until the crust is golden and the cheese is melted and bubbly.
8. Remove from the oven and let the pizza cool for a few minutes before slicing and serving.

Nutritional Information (per serving):
- Calories: 260 kcal
- Fat: 8g
- Carbohydrates: 30g
- Fiber: 6g
- Protein: 14g

10. Three Cheese Garden Delight

Intro: Three Cheese Garden Delight pizza is a cheesy delight featuring a blend of reduced-fat cheeses, fresh garden vegetables, and aromatic herbs on a whole wheat crust, offering a satisfying and flavorful meal option.

Total Time: 30 minutes

Servings: 4

Ingredients:
- 1 pre-made whole wheat pizza crust
- 1/2 cup tomato sauce
- 1 cup sliced bell peppers (red, green, and yellow)
- 1 cup sliced mushrooms
- 1/2 cup sliced red onion
- 1/2 cup sliced black olives
- 1/2 cup reduced-fat shredded mozzarella cheese
- 1/4 cup reduced-fat shredded cheddar cheese
- 1/4 cup reduced-fat shredded Parmesan cheese

- 1 tablespoon olive oil
- Salt and pepper to taste
- Italian seasoning (optional)

Directions:

1. Preheat your oven to 425°F (220°C).
2. Spread the tomato sauce evenly over the pizza crust.
3. Arrange the sliced bell peppers, mushrooms, red onion, and black olives on top of the sauce.
4. In a small bowl, mix together the reduced-fat shredded mozzarella, cheddar, and Parmesan cheeses.
5. Sprinkle the cheese mixture evenly over the vegetables.
6. Drizzle the olive oil over the toppings and season with salt, pepper, and Italian seasoning if desired.
7. Bake the pizza in the preheated oven for 15-20 minutes, or until the crust is golden and the cheese is melted and bubbly.
8. Remove from the oven and let the pizza cool for a few minutes before slicing and serving.

Nutritional Information (per serving):
- Calories: 280 kcal
- Fat: 11g
- Carbohydrates: 35g
- Fiber: 6g
- Protein: 14g

Enjoy these delicious and nutritious low-fat pizza recipes featuring a variety of low-fat cheese selections!

Chapter 7: Specialty low-fat pizza

1. Southwest Chicken Fiesta

Intro: Southwest Chicken Fiesta pizza brings the bold flavors of the Southwest to your plate with tender chicken, spicy salsa, black beans, and vibrant veggies atop a crispy crust.

Total Time: 30 minutes

Servings: 4

Ingredients:
- 1 pre-made whole wheat pizza crust
- 1/2 cup salsa
- 1 cup cooked chicken breast, shredded
- 1/2 cup black beans, drained and rinsed
- 1/2 cup corn kernels
- 1/2 cup diced bell peppers (red, green, and yellow)
- 1/4 cup diced red onion
- 1 cup reduced-fat shredded Mexican cheese blend
- 1 tablespoon chopped fresh cilantro (optional)
- Olive oil cooking spray

Directions:
1. Preheat your oven to 425°F (220°C).
2. Spray a baking sheet with olive oil cooking spray and place the pizza crust on it.
3. Spread the salsa evenly over the pizza crust.
4. Scatter the shredded chicken, black beans, corn kernels, bell peppers, and red onion over the salsa.
5. Sprinkle the reduced-fat shredded Mexican cheese blend over the toppings.

6. Bake the pizza in the preheated oven for 12-15 minutes, or until the crust is golden and the cheese is melted and bubbly.
7. Remove from the oven and let the pizza cool for a few minutes before slicing.
8. Garnish with chopped fresh cilantro, if desired, before serving.

Nutritional Information (per serving):
- Calories: 290 kcal
- Fat: 8g
- Carbohydrates: 35g
- Fiber: 6g
- Protein: 18g

2. Mediterranean Veggie Delight

Intro: Mediterranean Veggie Delight pizza transports your taste buds to the shores of the Mediterranean with a delightful combination of sun-dried tomatoes, artichoke hearts, olives, and feta cheese atop a crispy crust.

Total Time: 25 minutes

Servings: 4

Ingredients:
- 1 pre-made whole wheat pizza crust
- 1/2 cup tomato sauce
- 1/4 cup sliced sun-dried tomatoes
- 1/4 cup sliced artichoke hearts
- 1/4 cup sliced Kalamata olives
- 1/4 cup sliced black olives
- 1/2 cup reduced-fat crumbled feta cheese
- 1 tablespoon olive oil
- Salt and pepper to taste
- Fresh oregano leaves for garnish (optional)

Directions:
1. Preheat your oven to 425°F (220°C).
2. Spread the tomato sauce evenly over the pizza crust.
3. Scatter the sliced sun-dried tomatoes, artichoke hearts, Kalamata olives, and black olives over the sauce.
4. Sprinkle the reduced-fat crumbled feta cheese over the toppings.
5. Drizzle the olive oil over the pizza and season with salt and pepper to taste.

6. Bake the pizza in the preheated oven for 12-15 minutes, or until the crust is golden and the cheese is melted and bubbly.
7. Remove from the oven and let the pizza cool for a few minutes before slicing.
8. Garnish with fresh oregano leaves before serving, if desired.

Nutritional Information (per serving):
- Calories: 260 kcal
- Fat: 10g
- Carbohydrates: 30g
- Fiber: 6g
- Protein: 12g

3. Hawaiian BBQ Bliss

Intro: Hawaiian BBQ Bliss pizza brings the flavors of the tropics to your table with tender pieces of grilled chicken, sweet pineapple chunks, tangy barbecue sauce, and reduced-fat mozzarella cheese on a whole wheat crust.

Total Time: 30 minutes

Servings: 4

Ingredients:
- 1 pre-made whole wheat pizza crust
- 1/2 cup barbecue sauce (low-sugar, if available)
- 1 cup cooked chicken breast, shredded
- 1/2 cup pineapple chunks (fresh or canned, drained)
- 1/4 cup sliced red onion
- 1 cup reduced-fat shredded mozzarella cheese
- 1 tablespoon chopped fresh cilantro (optional)
- Olive oil cooking spray

Directions:
1. Preheat your oven to 425°F (220°C).
2. Spray a baking sheet with olive oil cooking spray and place the pizza crust on it.
3. Spread the barbecue sauce evenly over the pizza crust.
4. Scatter the shredded chicken, pineapple chunks, and sliced red onion over the barbecue sauce.

5. Sprinkle the reduced-fat shredded mozzarella cheese over the toppings.
6. Bake the pizza in the preheated oven for 12-15 minutes, or until the crust is golden and the cheese is melted and bubbly.
7. Remove from the oven and let the pizza cool for a few minutes before slicing.
8. Garnish with chopped fresh cilantro, if desired, before serving.

Nutritional Information (per serving):
- Calories: 280 kcal
- Fat: 8g
- Carbohydrates: 35g
- Fiber: 6g
- Protein: 18g

4. Thai Peanut Veggie Fusion

Intro: Thai Peanut Veggie Fusion pizza combines the exotic flavors of Thailand with an array of colorful vegetables, creamy peanut sauce, and reduced-fat cheese on a wholesome crust, offering a unique and delicious culinary experience.

Total Time: 25 minutes

Servings: 4

Ingredients:
- 1 pre-made whole wheat pizza crust
- 1/4 cup peanut sauce (store-bought or homemade)
- 1 cup sliced bell peppers (red, green, and yellow)
- 1 cup sliced carrots
- 1/2 cup sliced red cabbage
- 1/4 cup sliced green onions
- 1/2 cup reduced-fat shredded mozzarella cheese
- Crushed peanuts for garnish (optional)
- Fresh cilantro leaves for garnish (optional)

Directions:
1. Preheat your oven to 425°F (220°C).
2. Spread the peanut sauce evenly over the pizza crust.

3. Arrange the sliced bell peppers, carrots, red cabbage, and green onions on top of the sauce.
4. Sprinkle the reduced-fat shredded mozzarella cheese over the vegetables.
5. Bake the pizza in the preheated oven for 12-15 minutes, or until the crust is golden and the cheese is melted and bubbly.
6. Remove from the oven and let the pizza cool for a few minutes before slicing.
7. Garnish with crushed peanuts and fresh cilantro leaves, if desired, before serving.

Nutritional Information (per serving):
- Calories: 270 kcal
- Fat: 8g
- Carbohydrates: 30g
- Fiber: 6g
- Protein: 14

5. Buffalo Cauliflower Ranch

Intro: Buffalo Cauliflower Ranch pizza offers a vegetarian twist on the classic buffalo chicken pizza, featuring crispy roasted cauliflower florets tossed in spicy buffalo sauce, creamy ranch dressing, and reduced-fat cheese on a whole wheat crust.

Total Time: 35 minutes

Servings: 4

Ingredients:
- 1 pre-made whole wheat pizza crust
- 2 cups cauliflower florets
- 1/4 cup buffalo sauce
- 1/4 cup ranch dressing (low-fat, if available)
- 1/2 cup sliced red onion
- 1/2 cup sliced celery
- 1 cup reduced-fat shredded mozzarella cheese
- 1 tablespoon chopped fresh parsley (optional)
- Olive oil cooking spray

Directions:
1. Preheat your oven to 425°F (220°C).
2. Place the cauliflower florets on a baking sheet lined with parchment paper. Spray

with olive oil cooking spray and roast in the preheated oven for 20 minutes, or until crispy and lightly browned.

3. Remove the cauliflower from the oven and toss with buffalo sauce until evenly coated.
4. Spread the ranch dressing evenly over the pizza crust.
5. Scatter the buffalo cauliflower, sliced red onion, and sliced celery over the ranch dressing.
6. Sprinkle the reduced-fat shredded mozzarella cheese over the toppings.
7. Bake the pizza in the preheated oven for 12-15 minutes, or until the crust is golden and the cheese is melted and bubbly.
8. Remove from the oven and let the pizza cool for a few minutes before slicing.
9. Garnish with chopped fresh parsley, if desired, before serving.

Nutritional Information (per serving):
- Calories: 280 kcal
- Fat: 9g

- Carbohydrates: 35g
- Fiber: 6g
- Protein: 16g

6. Caprese Pesto Perfection

Intro: Caprese Pesto Perfection pizza is a delightful blend of ripe tomatoes, fresh basil, creamy mozzarella cheese, and aromatic pesto sauce on a whole wheat crust, capturing the essence of a classic Caprese salad in every bite.

Total Time: 25 minutes

Servings: 4

Ingredients:
- 1 pre-made whole wheat pizza crust
- 1/2 cup pesto sauce (store-bought or homemade)
- 1 cup sliced ripe tomatoes
- 1 cup fresh basil leaves
- 8 ounces fresh mozzarella cheese, thinly sliced
- 2 cloves garlic, minced
- 1 tablespoon olive oil
- Salt and pepper to taste

Directions:
1. Preheat your oven to 425°F (220°C).
2. Spread the minced garlic evenly over the pizza crust.
3. Arrange the sliced tomatoes on top of the garlic.
4. Place the fresh basil leaves on top of the tomatoes.
5. Arrange the slices of fresh mozzarella cheese over the basil leaves.
6. Drizzle the olive oil over the toppings and season with salt and pepper to taste.
7. Bake the pizza in the preheated oven for 12-15 minutes, or until the crust is golden and the cheese is melted and bubbly.
8. Remove from the oven and let the pizza cool for a few minutes before slicing and serving.

Nutritional Information (per serving):
- Calories: 290 kcal
- Fat: 13g
- Carbohydrates: 30g
- Fiber: 6g
- Protein: 12g

7. Taco Tuesday Supreme

Intro: Taco Tuesday Supreme pizza is a fiesta of flavors, featuring seasoned ground turkey, black beans, corn, bell peppers, and jalapeños, topped with reduced-fat cheese and served on a crispy whole wheat crust.

Total Time: 30 minutes

Servings: 4

Ingredients:
- 1 pre-made whole wheat pizza crust
- 1/2 cup salsa
- 1 cup cooked ground turkey (seasoned with taco seasoning)
- 1/2 cup black beans, drained and rinsed
- 1/2 cup corn kernels
- 1/2 cup diced bell peppers (red, green, and yellow)
- 1/4 cup sliced jalapeños (optional)
- 1 cup reduced-fat shredded Mexican cheese blend
- 1 tablespoon chopped fresh cilantro (optional)

- Olive oil cooking spray

Directions:
1. Preheat your oven to 425°F (220°C).
2. Spray a baking sheet with olive oil cooking spray and place the pizza crust on it.
3. Spread the salsa evenly over the pizza crust.
4. Scatter the cooked ground turkey, black beans, corn kernels, diced bell peppers, and sliced jalapeños over the salsa.
5. Sprinkle the reduced-fat shredded Mexican cheese blend over the toppings.
6. Bake the pizza in the preheated oven for 12-15 minutes, or until the crust is golden and the cheese is melted and bubbly.
7. Remove from the oven and let the pizza cool for a few minutes before slicing.
8. Garnish with chopped fresh cilantro, if desired, before serving.

Nutritional Information (per serving):
- Calories: 310 kcal
- Fat: 9g
- Carbohydrates: 35g

- Fiber: 6g
- Protein: 20g

8. Greek Gyro Sensation

Intro: Greek Gyro Sensation pizza offers a taste of the Mediterranean with seasoned lean ground beef, tzatziki sauce, tomatoes, red onions, and feta cheese on a whole wheat crust, delivering a satisfying and flavorful experience.

Total Time: 30 minutes

Servings: 4

Ingredients:
- 1 pre-made whole wheat pizza crust
- 1/2 cup tzatziki sauce
- 1 cup cooked lean ground beef (seasoned with Greek spices)
- 1/2 cup diced tomatoes
- 1/4 cup sliced red onions
- 1/4 cup sliced black olives
- 1/4 cup crumbled feta cheese
- Fresh dill for garnish (optional)
- Olive oil cooking spray

Directions:
1. Preheat your oven to 425°F (220°C).
2. Spray a baking sheet with olive oil cooking spray and place the pizza crust on it.
3. Spread the tzatziki sauce evenly over the pizza crust.
4. Scatter the cooked lean ground beef, diced tomatoes, sliced red onions, and sliced black olives over the tzatziki sauce.
5. Sprinkle the crumbled feta cheese over the toppings.
6. Bake the pizza in the preheated oven for 12-15 minutes, or until the crust is golden and the cheese is melted and bubbly.
7. Remove from the oven and let the pizza cool for a few minutes before slicing.
8. Garnish with fresh dill, if desired, before serving.

Nutritional Information (per serving):
- Calories: 300 kcal
- Fat: 10g
- Carbohydrates: 35g
- Fiber: 6g

- Protein: 18g

9. Teriyaki Tofu Temptation

Intro: Teriyaki Tofu Temptation pizza offers a delightful fusion of Asian flavors, featuring marinated tofu, colorful bell peppers, pineapple chunks, and a tangy teriyaki sauce on a whole wheat crust, creating a satisfying and flavorful meal option.

Total Time: 35 minutes

Servings: 4

Ingredients:
- 1 pre-made whole wheat pizza crust
- 1/2 cup teriyaki sauce (low-sodium, if available)
- 1 cup extra-firm tofu, pressed and cubed
- 1/2 cup diced bell peppers (red, green, and yellow)
- 1/2 cup pineapple chunks (fresh or canned, drained)
- 1/4 cup sliced red onion
- 1 cup reduced-fat shredded mozzarella cheese

- 1 tablespoon chopped green onions for garnish (optional)
- Olive oil cooking spray

Directions:

1. Preheat your oven to 425°F (220°C).
2. Spray a baking sheet with olive oil cooking spray and place the pizza crust on it.
3. Spread the teriyaki sauce evenly over the pizza crust.
4. Arrange the cubed tofu, diced bell peppers, pineapple chunks, and sliced red onion over the teriyaki sauce.
5. Sprinkle the reduced-fat shredded mozzarella cheese over the toppings.
6. Bake the pizza in the preheated oven for 15-20 minutes, or until the crust is golden and the cheese is melted and bubbly.
7. Remove from the oven and let the pizza cool for a few minutes before slicing.
8. Garnish with chopped green onions, if desired, before serving.

Nutritional Information (per serving):

- Calories: 280 kcal
- Fat: 9g

- Carbohydrates: 30g
- Fiber: 6g
- Protein: 16g

10. BBQ Pulled Pork Paradise

Intro: BBQ Pulled Pork Paradise pizza offers a savory twist on traditional barbecue flavors, featuring tender pulled pork, tangy barbecue sauce, red onions, and cilantro atop a whole wheat crust, creating a mouthwatering and satisfying dish.

Total Time: 35 minutes

Servings: 4

Ingredients:
- 1 pre-made whole wheat pizza crust
- 1/2 cup barbecue sauce (low-sugar, if available)
- 1 cup cooked pulled pork
- 1/4 cup sliced red onions
- 1/4 cup chopped fresh cilantro
- 1 cup reduced-fat shredded mozzarella cheese
- Olive oil cooking spray

Directions:
1. Preheat your oven to 425°F (220°C).
2. Spray a baking sheet with olive oil cooking spray and place the pizza crust on it.
3. Spread the barbecue sauce evenly over the pizza crust.
4. Scatter the cooked pulled pork and sliced red onions over the barbecue sauce.
5. Sprinkle the reduced-fat shredded mozzarella cheese over the toppings.
6. Bake the pizza in the preheated oven for 15-20 minutes, or until the crust is golden and the cheese is melted and bubbly.
7. Remove from the oven and let the pizza cool for a few minutes before slicing.
8. Garnish with chopped fresh cilantro before serving.

Nutritional Information (per serving):
- Calories: 290 kcal
- Fat: 10g
- Carbohydrates: 30g
- Fiber: 6g
- Protein: 18g

Enjoy these specialty low-fat pizza recipes bursting with unique flavors and wholesome ingredients!

Chapter 8: Low-fat dessert pizza

1. Apple Cinnamon Delight

Intro: Apple Cinnamon Delight pizza is a comforting dessert featuring sweet apple slices, fragrant cinnamon, and a hint of brown sugar on a crispy crust, making it a delightful treat for any occasion.

Total Time: 30 minutes

Servings: 4

Ingredients:
- 1 pre-made whole wheat pizza crust
- 2 medium apples, thinly sliced
- 1 tablespoon lemon juice
- 1 teaspoon ground cinnamon
- 2 tablespoons brown sugar (or sweetener of choice)
- 2 tablespoons reduced-fat cream cheese
- 1 tablespoon honey
- 1 tablespoon chopped walnuts (optional)

Directions:

1. Preheat your oven to 425°F (220°C).
2. In a bowl, toss the thinly sliced apples with lemon juice, cinnamon, and brown sugar until evenly coated.
3. Spread the reduced-fat cream cheese evenly over the pizza crust.
4. Arrange the apple slices in a single layer over the cream cheese.
5. Drizzle honey over the apples.
6. Sprinkle chopped walnuts over the top, if using.
7. Bake the pizza in the preheated oven for 15-20 minutes, or until the crust is golden and the apples are tender.
8. Remove from the oven and let the pizza cool for a few minutes before slicing.
9. Serve warm and enjoy!

Nutritional Information (per serving):

- Calories: 220 kcal
- Fat: 5g
- Carbohydrates: 40g
- Fiber: 6g
- Protein: 4g

2. Berry Blast Sweetness

Intro: Berry Blast Sweetness pizza is a burst of fruity flavors with a combination of fresh berries, a drizzle of honey, and a sprinkle of mint leaves on a light and crispy crust, offering a refreshing and guilt-free dessert option.

Total Time: 25 minutes

Servings: 4

Ingredients:
- 1 pre-made whole wheat pizza crust
- 1 cup mixed berries (such as strawberries, blueberries, raspberries)
- 2 tablespoons honey
- Fresh mint leaves for garnish
- Reduced-fat whipped cream or Greek yogurt (optional)

Directions:
1. Preheat your oven to 425°F (220°C).
2. Place the pizza crust on a baking sheet.
3. Arrange the mixed berries evenly over the pizza crust.
4. Drizzle honey over the berries.

5. Bake the pizza in the preheated oven for 10-12 minutes, or until the crust is golden and the berries are slightly softened.
6. Remove from the oven and let the pizza cool for a few minutes.
7. Garnish with fresh mint leaves.
8. Serve warm, optionally topped with a dollop of reduced-fat whipped cream or Greek yogurt.

Nutritional Information (per serving):
- Calories: 160 kcal
- Fat: 1g
- Carbohydrates: 35g
- Fiber: 6g
- Protein: 3g

3. Chocolate Banana Dream

Intro: Chocolate Banana Dream pizza is a decadent dessert featuring creamy chocolate spread, sweet banana slices, and a sprinkle of toasted almonds on a golden crust, creating a heavenly treat for chocolate lovers.

Low Fat Pizza Recipes

Total Time: 20 minutes
Servings: 4

Ingredients:
- 1 pre-made whole wheat pizza crust
- 1/4 cup chocolate spread (low-fat, if available)
- 2 ripe bananas, thinly sliced
- 2 tablespoons toasted sliced almonds
- Powdered sugar for dusting (optional)

Directions:
1. Preheat your oven to 425°F (220°C).
2. Place the pizza crust on a baking sheet.
3. Spread the chocolate spread evenly over the pizza crust.
4. Arrange the thinly sliced bananas over the chocolate spread.
5. Sprinkle the toasted sliced almonds over the bananas.
6. Bake the pizza in the preheated oven for 10-12 minutes, or until the crust is golden and the chocolate is melted.
7. Remove from the oven and let the pizza cool for a few minutes.
8. Dust with powdered sugar, if desired, before serving.

Nutritional Information (per serving):
- Calories: 210 kcal
- Fat: 6g
- Carbohydrates: 35g
- Fiber: 6g
- Protein: 4g

4. Tropical Fruit Paradise

Intro: Tropical Fruit Paradise pizza is a taste of the tropics, featuring a medley of tropical fruits such as mango, pineapple, and kiwi, drizzled with a tangy citrus glaze on a crispy crust, offering a refreshing and exotic dessert experience.

Total Time: 30 minutes

Servings: 4

Ingredients:
- 1 pre-made whole wheat pizza crust
- 1 mango, peeled and diced
- 1 cup diced pineapple
- 2 kiwi, peeled and sliced
- 2 tablespoons orange juice

- 1 tablespoon honey
- Shredded coconut for garnish (optional)
- Fresh mint leaves for garnish (optional)

Directions:
1. Preheat your oven to 425°F (220°C).
2. Place the pizza crust on a baking sheet.
3. Arrange the diced mango, pineapple, and sliced kiwi evenly over the pizza crust.
4. In a small bowl, whisk together the orange juice and honey to make the citrus glaze.
5. Drizzle the citrus glaze over the fruits on the pizza.
6. Bake the pizza in the preheated oven for 10-12 minutes, or until the crust is golden and the fruits are slightly caramelized.
7. Remove from the oven and let the pizza cool for a few minutes.
8. Garnish with shredded coconut and fresh mint leaves, if desired, before serving.

Nutritional Information (per serving):
- Calories: 180 kcal

- Fat: 2g
- Carbohydrates: 40g
- Fiber: 6g
- Protein: 3g

5. Peanut Butter Cup Pleasure

Intro: Peanut Butter Cup Pleasure pizza is a delightful dessert that combines the creamy richness of peanut butter with the sweetness of chocolate chips, all melted on a warm, crispy crust, creating a comforting and indulgent treat.

Total Time: 15 minutes

Servings: 4

Ingredients:
- 1 pre-made whole wheat pizza crust
- 1/2 cup creamy peanut butter (low-fat, if available)
- 1/4 cup chocolate chips (semi-sweet or dark)
- 2 tablespoons honey or maple syrup
- Sliced bananas for topping (optional)

Directions:

1. Preheat your oven to 425°F (220°C).
2. Place the pizza crust on a baking sheet.
3. Spread the creamy peanut butter evenly over the pizza crust.
4. Sprinkle the chocolate chips over the peanut butter.
5. Drizzle honey or maple syrup over the toppings.
6. Bake the pizza in the preheated oven for 8-10 minutes, or until the crust is golden and the chocolate is melted.
7. Remove from the oven and let the pizza cool for a few minutes.
8. Optionally, top with sliced bananas before serving.

Nutritional Information (per serving):
- Calories: 320 kcal
- Fat: 18g
- Carbohydrates: 30g
- Fiber: 4g
- Protein: 10g

6. Lemon Berry Bliss

Intro: Lemon Berry Bliss pizza is a refreshing and zesty dessert featuring a tangy lemon curd spread, topped with a medley of fresh berries and a sprinkle of powdered sugar on a crispy crust, offering a burst of summer flavors.

Total Time: 25 minutes

Servings: 4

Ingredients:
- 1 pre-made whole wheat pizza crust
- 1/2 cup lemon curd (low-fat, if available)
- 1 cup mixed berries (such as strawberries, blueberries, raspberries)
- Powdered sugar for dusting
- Lemon zest for garnish (optional)

Directions:
1. Preheat your oven to 425°F (220°C).
2. Place the pizza crust on a baking sheet.
3. Spread the lemon curd evenly over the pizza crust.
4. Arrange the mixed berries over the lemon curd.
5. Bake the pizza in the preheated oven for 10-12 minutes, or until the crust is golden and the berries are slightly softened.

6. Remove from the oven and let the pizza cool for a few minutes.
7. Dust with powdered sugar before serving.
8. Garnish with lemon zest, if desired.

Nutritional Information (per serving):

- Calories: 250 kcal
- Fat: 6g
- Carbohydrates: 45g
- Fiber: 6g
- Protein: 4g

7. Caramel Apple Crisp

Intro: Caramel Apple Crisp pizza is a comforting dessert reminiscent of classic apple crisp, featuring tender apple slices, a sprinkle of cinnamon, crunchy granola topping, and a drizzle of caramel sauce on a golden crust, offering a delightful blend of flavors and textures.

Total Time: 35 minutes

Servings: 4

Low Fat Pizza Recipes

Ingredients:
- 1 pre-made whole wheat pizza crust
- 2 medium apples, thinly sliced
- 1 tablespoon lemon juice
- 1 teaspoon ground cinnamon
- 1/2 cup granola
- 2 tablespoons caramel sauce (low-fat, if available)
- Reduced-fat vanilla ice cream for serving (optional)

Directions:
1. Preheat your oven to 425°F (220°C).
2. Place the pizza crust on a baking sheet.
3. In a bowl, toss the thinly sliced apples with lemon juice and ground cinnamon until evenly coated.
4. Arrange the apple slices over the pizza crust.
5. Sprinkle granola evenly over the apples.
6. Bake the pizza in the preheated oven for 20-25 minutes, or until the apples are tender and the crust is golden.
7. Remove from the oven and let the pizza cool for a few minutes.
8. Drizzle caramel sauce over the pizza before serving.

9. Serve warm, optionally topped with reduced-fat vanilla ice cream.

Nutritional Information (per serving):
- Calories: 280 kcal
- Fat: 5g
- Carbohydrates: 55g
- Fiber: 7g
- Protein: 4g

8. Nutella Strawberry Sensation

Intro: Nutella Strawberry Sensation pizza is a heavenly dessert featuring creamy Nutella spread, fresh strawberry slices, and a dusting of powdered sugar on a warm, crispy crust, creating a blissful combination of chocolate and strawberries.

Total Time: 20 minutes

Servings: 4

Ingredients:
- 1 pre-made whole wheat pizza crust

- 1/2 cup Nutella or hazelnut chocolate spread
- 1 cup fresh strawberries, hulled and sliced
- Powdered sugar for dusting
- Fresh mint leaves for garnish (optional)

Directions:

1. Preheat your oven to 425°F (220°C).
2. Place the pizza crust on a baking sheet.
3. Spread the Nutella evenly over the pizza crust.
4. Arrange the sliced strawberries over the Nutella.
5. Bake the pizza in the preheated oven for 8-10 minutes, or until the crust is golden and the Nutella is melted.
6. Remove from the oven and let the pizza cool for a few minutes.
7. Dust with powdered sugar before serving.
8. Garnish with fresh mint leaves, if desired.

Nutritional Information (per serving):

- Calories: 310 kcal
- Fat: 12g
- Carbohydrates: 45g

- Fiber: 4g
- Protein: 4g

9. Peach Melba Delight

Intro: Peach Melba Delight pizza is a delightful dessert inspired by the classic Peach Melba dessert, featuring sweet peach slices, tangy raspberry sauce, and a sprinkle of almond slices on a golden crust, offering a taste of summer in every bite.

Total Time: 30 minutes

Servings: 4

Ingredients:
- 1 pre-made whole wheat pizza crust
- 2 ripe peaches, thinly sliced
- 1/2 cup raspberry sauce (low-sugar, if available)
- 2 tablespoons sliced almonds
- Fresh raspberries for garnish (optional)
- Fresh mint leaves for garnish (optional)

Directions:
1. Preheat your oven to 425°F (220°C).
2. Place the pizza crust on a baking sheet.
3. Arrange the thinly sliced peaches over the pizza crust.
4. Drizzle raspberry sauce evenly over the peaches.
5. Sprinkle sliced almonds over the top.
6. Bake the pizza in the preheated oven for 10-12 minutes, or until the crust is golden and the peaches are tender.
7. Remove from the oven and let the pizza cool for a few minutes.
8. Garnish with fresh raspberries and mint leaves, if desired, before serving.

Nutritional Information (per serving):
- Calories: 230 kcal
- Fat: 5g
- Carbohydrates: 40g
- Fiber: 6g
- Protein: 4g

10. Almond Joy Indulgence

Intro: Almond Joy Indulgence pizza is a decadent dessert inspired by the popular candy bar, featuring a luscious combination of chocolate spread, toasted coconut flakes, crunchy almonds, and a drizzle of caramel sauce on a warm, crispy crust, offering a delightful treat for chocolate and coconut lovers.

Total Time: 20 minutes

Servings: 4

Ingredients:
- 1 pre-made whole wheat pizza crust
- 1/4 cup chocolate spread (low-fat, if available)
- 1/4 cup shredded coconut, toasted
- 2 tablespoons sliced almonds, toasted
- 2 tablespoons caramel sauce (low-fat, if available)

Directions:
1. Preheat your oven to 425°F (220°C).
2. Place the pizza crust on a baking sheet.

3. Spread the chocolate spread evenly over the pizza crust.
4. Sprinkle toasted shredded coconut and sliced almonds over the chocolate spread.
5. Drizzle caramel sauce over the top.
6. Bake the pizza in the preheated oven for 8-10 minutes, or until the crust is golden and the toppings are heated through.
7. Remove from the oven and let the pizza cool for a few minutes.
8. Slice and serve warm.

Nutritional Information (per serving):
- Calories: 280 kcal
- Fat: 12g
- Carbohydrates: 40g
- Fiber: 6g
- Protein: 4g

Enjoy these delightful low-fat dessert pizzas that are perfect for satisfying your sweet cravings without the guilt!

Chapter 9: Low-fat pizza Sides and Dips

1. Garlic Parmesan Zucchini Fries

Intro: Garlic Parmesan Zucchini Fries are a delicious alternative to traditional fries, offering a crispy texture with a burst of garlic and Parmesan flavor.

Total Time: 25 minutes

Servings: 4

Ingredients:
- 2 medium zucchinis, cut into fries
- 1/4 cup whole wheat breadcrumbs
- 2 tablespoons grated Parmesan cheese
- 1 teaspoon garlic powder
- 1/2 teaspoon dried oregano
- Salt and pepper to taste
- Olive oil cooking spray

Directions:

1. Preheat the oven to 425°F (220°C) and line a baking sheet with parchment paper.
2. In a bowl, combine breadcrumbs, Parmesan cheese, garlic powder, oregano, salt, and pepper.
3. Dip each zucchini fry into the breadcrumb mixture, ensuring it's evenly coated, and place it on the prepared baking sheet.
4. Lightly spray the zucchini fries with olive oil cooking spray.
5. Bake for 15-20 minutes, flipping halfway through, until the fries are golden brown and crispy.
6. Serve hot with your favorite dipping sauce.

Nutritional Information (per serving):

- Calories: 70 kcal
- Fat: 2g
- Carbohydrates: 10g
- Fiber: 2g
- Protein: 4g

2. Greek Yogurt Ranch Dip

Intro: Greek Yogurt Ranch Dip is a healthier twist on the classic ranch dip, packed with protein and tangy flavors, perfect for dipping veggies or spreading on pizza crusts.

Total Time: 5 minutes

Servings: 8

Ingredients:
- 1 cup plain Greek yogurt
- 1 tablespoon dried parsley
- 1 teaspoon dried dill
- 1 teaspoon garlic powder
- 1 teaspoon onion powder
- 1/2 teaspoon dried chives
- Salt and pepper to taste

Directions:
1. In a bowl, mix together Greek yogurt, dried parsley, dried dill, garlic powder, onion powder, dried chives, salt, and pepper until well combined.
2. Adjust seasoning to taste.

3. Serve immediately or refrigerate for at least 30 minutes to allow flavors to meld.
4. Serve with veggie sticks, pizza slices, or as a spread for pizza crusts.

Nutritional Information (per serving):
- Calories: 25 kcal
- Fat: 0g
- Carbohydrates: 2g
- Fiber: 0g
- Protein: 3g

3. Balsamic Glazed Brussels Sprouts

Intro: Balsamic Glazed Brussels Sprouts offer a delightful combination of sweet and tangy flavors, making them a perfect side dish or appetizer to complement your low-fat pizza.

Total Time: 20 minutes

Servings: 4

Ingredients:
- 1pound Brussels sprouts, trimmed and halved

- 2 tablespoons balsamic vinegar
- 1 tablespoon honey
- 1 tablespoon olive oil
- Salt and pepper to taste

Directions:

1. Preheat the oven to 400°F (200°C) and line a baking sheet with parchment paper.
2. In a bowl, whisk together balsamic vinegar, honey, olive oil, salt, and pepper.
3. Add Brussels sprouts to the bowl and toss until they are evenly coated with the balsamic mixture.
4. Spread the Brussels sprouts in a single layer on the prepared baking sheet.
5. Roast in the preheated oven for 15-20 minutes, or until they are tender and caramelized, stirring halfway through.
6. Remove from the oven and serve immediately as a side dish or appetizer.

Nutritional Information (per serving):
- Calories: 70 kcal
- Fat: 3g

- Carbohydrates: 10g
- Fiber: 3g
- Protein: 3g

4. Caprese Salad Skewers

Intro: Caprese Salad Skewers are a fresh and flavorful appetizer or side dish featuring cherry tomatoes, mozzarella balls, and fresh basil leaves drizzled with balsamic glaze, creating a colorful and delicious addition to your meal.

Total Time: 15 minutes

Servings: 4

Ingredients:
- 1 cup cherry tomatoes
- 1 cup mini mozzarella balls
- Fresh basil leaves
- Balsamic glaze for drizzling

Directions:
1. Thread cherry tomatoes, mini mozzarella balls, and fresh basil leaves

onto skewers, alternating the ingredients.

2. Arrange the skewers on a serving platter.
3. Drizzle balsamic glaze over the skewers just before serving.
4. Enjoy immediately as a refreshing side dish or appetizer.

Nutritional Information (per serving):
- Calories: 90 kcal
- Fat: 6g
- Carbohydrates: 3g
- Fiber: 1g
- Protein: 7g

5. Roasted Red Pepper Hummus

Intro: Roasted Red Pepper Hummus is a creamy and flavorful dip made with chickpeas, roasted red peppers, tahini, garlic, and lemon juice, perfect for dipping pizza crusts or serving alongside your favorite low-fat pizza.

Total Time: 15 minutes

Servings: 8

Ingredients:
- 1 can (15 ounces) chickpeas, drained and rinsed
- 1/2 cup roasted red peppers, drained
- 2 tablespoons tahini
- 2 cloves garlic, minced
- 2 tablespoons lemon juice
- 2 tablespoons olive oil
- Salt and pepper to taste
- Paprika for garnish (optional)
- Chopped fresh parsley for garnish (optional)

Directions:
1. In a food processor, combine chickpeas, roasted red peppers, tahini, garlic, lemon juice, olive oil, salt, and pepper.
2. Blend until smooth and creamy, scraping down the sides as needed.
3. Taste and adjust seasoning as desired.
4. Transfer the hummus to a serving bowl.
5. Garnish with a sprinkle of paprika and chopped fresh parsley, if desired.
6. Serve with pizza crusts or vegetable sticks for dipping.

Nutritional Information (per serving):
- Calories: 120 kcal
- Fat: 6g
- Carbohydrates: 12g
- Fiber: 3g
- Protein: 4g

6. Spinach and Artichoke Dip

Intro: Spinach and Artichoke Dip is a creamy and savory dip made with spinach, artichokes, Greek yogurt, and cheese, perfect for spreading on pizza crusts or dipping with breadsticks.

Total Time: 25 minutes

Servings: 8

Ingredients:
- 1 cup frozen chopped spinach, thawed and drained
- 1 can (14 ounces) artichoke hearts, drained and chopped
- 1 cup plain Greek yogurt
- 1/2 cup grated Parmesan cheese

- 1/2 cup shredded mozzarella cheese
- 2 cloves garlic, minced
- Salt and pepper to taste
- Olive oil cooking spray

Directions:

1. Preheat the oven to 375°F (190°C) and lightly grease a baking dish with olive oil cooking spray.
2. In a large bowl, mix together chopped spinach, chopped artichoke hearts, Greek yogurt, Parmesan cheese, mozzarella cheese, minced garlic, salt, and pepper.
3. Spread the mixture evenly into the prepared baking dish.
4. Bake in the preheated oven for 20-25 minutes, or until the dip is bubbly and lightly browned on top.
5. Remove from the oven and let it cool for a few minutes before serving.
6. Serve warm with pizza crusts or breadsticks for dipping.

Nutritional Information (per serving):

- Calories: 100 kcal
- Fat: 5g

- Carbohydrates: 6g
- Fiber: 2g
- Protein: 8g

7. Tomato Basil Bruschetta

Intro: Tomato Basil Bruschetta is a classic Italian appetizer featuring diced tomatoes, fresh basil, garlic, and balsamic vinegar served on toasted whole wheat bread slices, offering a burst of flavor and freshness.

Total Time: 15 minutes

Servings: 4

Ingredients:
- 2 cups diced tomatoes
- 1/4 cup chopped fresh basil leaves
- 2 cloves garlic, minced
- 1 tablespoon balsamic vinegar
- 1 tablespoon olive oil
- Salt and pepper to taste
- 4 slices whole wheat bread, toasted

Directions:

1. In a bowl, combine diced tomatoes, chopped basil leaves, minced garlic, balsamic vinegar, olive oil, salt, and pepper.
2. Mix well until all ingredients are evenly distributed.
3. Let the mixture sit for 5-10 minutes to allow the flavors to meld.
4. Spoon the tomato mixture onto the toasted whole wheat bread slices.
5. Serve immediately as an appetizer or side dish with your low-fat pizza.

Nutritional Information (per serving):
- Calories: 120 kcal
- Fat: 4g
- Carbohydrates: 18g
- Fiber: 3g
- Protein: 4g

8. Lemon Garlic Edamame

Intro: Lemon Garlic Edamame is a flavorful and nutritious side dish featuring steamed edamame tossed with zesty lemon juice, minced garlic, and a sprinkle of sea salt, offering a satisfying accompaniment to your low-fat pizza.

Total Time: 10 minutes

Servings: 4

Ingredients:
- 2 cups frozen edamame (in pods)
- 2 cloves garlic, minced
- 2 tablespoons lemon juice
- 1 tablespoon olive oil
- Sea salt to taste

Directions:
1. Cook the frozen edamame according to package instructions, usually by boiling or steaming, until tender.
2. Drain the cooked edamame and transfer them to a bowl.
3. In a small skillet, heat olive oil over medium heat. Add minced garlic and sauté for 1-2 minutes, until fragrant.
4. Pour the garlic-infused olive oil over the cooked edamame.
5. Add lemon juice and sea salt to taste. Toss to coat evenly.
6. Serve warm as a side dish with your low-fat pizza.

Nutritional Information (per serving):
- Calories: 120 kcal
- Fat: 6g
- Carbohydrates: 9g
- Fiber: 5g
- Protein: 9g

9. Cucumber Avocado Salad

Intro: Cucumber Avocado Salad is a refreshing and nutritious side dish featuring crisp cucumber slices, creamy avocado chunks, cherry tomatoes, and red onion tossed in a tangy vinaigrette, providing a burst of flavor and texture.

Total Time: 15 minutes

Servings: 4

Ingredients:
- 2 medium cucumbers, thinly sliced
- 1 ripe avocado, diced
- 1 cup cherry tomatoes, halved

- 1/4 cup thinly sliced red onion
- 2 tablespoons chopped fresh parsley
- 2 tablespoons olive oil
- 1 tablespoon lemon juice
- Salt and pepper to taste

Directions:

1. In a large bowl, combine cucumber slices, diced avocado, cherry tomatoes, sliced red onion, and chopped fresh parsley.
2. In a small bowl, whisk together olive oil, lemon juice, salt, and pepper to make the vinaigrette.
3. Pour the vinaigrette over the salad ingredients and toss gently to coat.
4. Serve immediately as a refreshing side dish with your low-fat pizza.

Nutritional Information (per serving):

- Calories: 150 kcal
- Fat: 12g
- Carbohydrates: 10g
- Fiber: 5g
- Protein: 2g

10. Honey Mustard Dipping Sauce

Intro: Honey Mustard Dipping Sauce is a sweet and tangy condiment perfect for dipping pizza crusts or serving alongside your favorite low-fat pizza, made with a combination of honey, Dijon mustard, Greek yogurt, and a splash of lemon juice.

Total Time: 5 minutes

Servings: 4

Ingredients:
- 1/4 cup Greek yogurt
- 2 tablespoons Dijon mustard
- 1 tablespoon honey
- 1 teaspoon lemon juice
- Salt and pepper to taste

Directions:
1. In a small bowl, whisk together Greek yogurt, Dijon mustard, honey, lemon juice, salt, and pepper until smooth and well combined.
2. Taste and adjust seasoning as desired.
3. Serve immediately as a dipping sauce with pizza crusts or breadsticks.

Nutritional Information (per serving):
- Calories: 30 kcal
- Fat: 0g
- Carbohydrates: 6g
- Fiber: 0g
- Protein: 2g

Enjoy these flavorful and healthy low-fat pizza sides and dips to elevate your pizza night! generate write up on

Chapter 10: Tips for Healthy Pizza Dining Out

Pizza dining out can be a delightful experience without compromising your health goals. By making informed choices and adopting smart strategies, you can enjoy your favorite pizza while staying mindful of your nutritional needs. In this chapter, we'll explore essential tips for navigating menus, making smart ingredient substitutions, and implementing portion control strategies to make your pizza dining experience healthier and more satisfying.

10.1 Navigating the Menu

When dining out for pizza, navigating the menu can often feel overwhelming with numerous options available.

To make healthier choices, consider the following tips:

- **Look for Whole Wheat Crust Options:** choose for whole wheat or whole grain crusts instead of refined flour options. Whole wheat crusts are higher in fiber and nutrients, making them a healthier choice.

- **Choose Lean Protein Toppings:** Select lean protein toppings such as grilled chicken, turkey sausage, or lean beef. These options provide protein without adding excess saturated fat and calories.

- **Load Up on Veggies:** Load your pizza with a variety of colorful vegetables such as bell peppers, mushrooms, onions, spinach, and tomatoes. Vegetables add flavor, texture, and essential nutrients to your pizza without significantly increasing calorie intake.

- **Watch Out for High-Calorie Toppings:** Be mindful of high-calorie toppings such as pepperoni, sausage, bacon, and extra cheese. While delicious, these toppings can quickly add up in calories, saturated fat, and sodium.

- **Consider Customizing Your Order:** Many pizza restaurants offer customization options. Don't hesitate to ask for adjustments to suit your preferences, such as less cheese, extra veggies, or a lighter cheese blend.

10.2 Making Smart Ingredient Substitutions

Making smart ingredient substitutions can significantly impact the nutritional profile of your pizza.

Here are some ideas for healthier swaps:

- **Choose Low-Fat Cheese:** Choose low-fat or part-skim cheese options instead of full-fat varieties. These alternatives provide similar flavor and texture with fewer calories and less saturated fat.

- **Use Lighter Sauce Options:** Look for pizzas with lighter sauce options such as marinara or tomato-based sauces instead of creamy or Alfredo sauces. Tomato-based sauces are lower in calories and fat while still adding flavor.

- **Explore Plant-Based Options:** Experiment with plant-based alternatives such as vegan cheese, tofu, or tempeh as protein sources. These options are often lower in saturated fat and cholesterol compared to animal-based proteins.

- **Swap Traditional Crust for Cauliflower Crust:** Some restaurants offer cauliflower crust as a gluten-free and lower-carb alternative. Cauliflower crusts are typically lower in calories and carbohydrates, making them suitable for those watching their intake of these nutrients.

10.3 Portion Control Strategies

Practicing portion control is key to enjoying pizza while managing your calorie intake.
Here are some portion control strategies to consider:

- **Share with Others:** Consider sharing a pizza with friends or family members to split the calories and prevent overeating.

- **Order a Small Size:** Go for a smaller pizza size or personal-sized pizza instead of a large or extra-large option. Smaller portions naturally limit calorie intake.

- **Pair with a Salad:** Accompany your pizza with a side salad loaded with leafy greens and vegetables. The fiber and volume from the salad can help increase satiety and reduce the urge to overindulge in pizza.

- **Box Half of Your Pizza:** If ordering a larger pizza, immediately box half of it to take home before starting your meal.

This prevents mindless eating and allows for portion control.

By implementing these tips for healthy pizza dining out, you can savor your favorite slices guilt-free while maintaining a balanced and nutritious diet. Enjoy your pizza experience while prioritizing your health and wellness goals!

www.ingramcontent.com/pod-product-compliance
Lightning Source LLC
Chambersburg PA
CBHW051610250726

48653CB00004BA/1443